The Nurse Anesthetist
and the Law

The Nurse Anesthetist and the Law

Mary Jeanette Mannino, C.R.N.A., J.D.

Principal Nurse Anesthetist
Assistant Clinical Professor, Anesthesiology
California College of Medicine
University of California, Irvine
Orange, California

Grune & Stratton
A Subsidiary of Harcourt Brace Jovanovich, Publishers
New York   London
Paris   San Diego   San Francisco   São Paulo
Sydney   Tokyo   Toronto

This publication is designed to provide accurate and authoritative information in regard to the subject matter covered. It is not intended to replace competent legal advice and is sold with the understanding that the publisher is not engaged in rendering legal or other professional services.

Library of Congress Cataloging in Publication Data

Mannino, Mary Jeannette.
    The nurse anesthetist and the law.

    Includes bibliographical references and index.
    1. Nurse anesthetists—Legal status, laws, etc.—United States. 2. Medical laws and legislation—United States. I. Title. [DNLM: 1. Nurse anesthetists—Legislation. WY 33.1 M284n]
KF2915.N8M36 1982   344.73'0414   82-11873
ISBN 0-8089-1496-0   347.304414

© 1982 by Grune & Stratton, Inc.
All rights reserved. No part of this publication
may be reproduced or transmitted in any form or
by any means, electronic or mechanical, including
photocopy, recording, or any information storage
and retrieval system, without permission in
writing from the publisher.

Grune & Stratton, Inc.
111 Fifth Avenue
New York, New York 10003

Distributed in the United Kingdom by
Academic Press Inc. (London) Ltd.
24/28 Oval Road, London NW 1

Library of Congress Catalog Number 82-11873
International Standard Book Number 0-8089-1496-0

Printed in the United States of America

To my parents

Contents

Acknowledgments   ix

Foreword   *Linda C. Larson*   xi

1. Legal History of Nurse Anesthesia   1
2. American Legal System   5
3. Statutory and Regulatory Law   13
4. Consent Law   31
5. Negligence   39
6. Anesthesia Practice and Lawsuits   59
7. Vicarious Liability   83
8. Employment Law   93
9. Anesthesia—Legal Cases   105

Glossary of Legal Terms   121

Appendixes
    A. Statute of Limitations   127

B. Basic Structure of the Union Contract: A Sample Outline   130

C. Sample Employment Agreement between Group Practice and C.R.N.A. Employee   142

D. Sample Employment Agreement between Hospital and Independent Contractor C.R.N.A.   145

E. Sample Employment Agreement between Hospital and Employee C.R.N.A.   149

F. Sample Employment Agreement between Hospital and Group Practice of which C.R.N.A. Is an Employee   152

Case Index   157

Index   165

Acknowledgments

As a courtroom observer in a malpractice case where one of the defendants was a nurse anesthetist, I became fully aware of the fact that although I had a good knowledge of anesthesia and the role of nurse anesthetists in the field, I possessed limited information on the legal aspects of the profession. My questions focused on why this anesthetist, one of the best I had ever worked with, was being made to explain her professional activities before a jury of lay people, who probably didn't know the difference between thiopental and nitrous oxide.

These and other questions persisted until I obtained a legal education. The legal process and its relation to nurse anesthesia have not been clearly defined, and I saw their definition as a job I could undertake.

There were many individuals who helped me work toward defining the relation of the legal process to nurse anesthesia. They are my friends and colleagues who supported me as I tried to combine legal research and writing with a busy anesthesia practice in a university hospital.

Although they are too numerous to name individually, I would like to thank as a group the certified registered nurse anesthetists employed at the University of California Irvine Medical Center. They exemplify the high practice standards and professionalism that prove nurse anesthesia is a significant force in the health care community. I particularly want to express thanks to A. Roselyn Wright and Dee Tuxen, who willingly helped me by covering my call duties and provided their moral support when I most needed it.

The faculty in the Department of Anesthesia, University of California, Irvine Medical College, deserve a word of thanks. Bruce F. Cullen, Chairman, and Dr. Richard Heyendal, Clinical Director, were particularly supportive in helping me with this project.

Friends and faculty from Irvine University School of Law deserve acknowledgment for their support. Included are Tim Stafford, J.D., who tolerated an anesthetist in his Law-Medicine class, and Marcia DeMarr, a true friend and classmate.

John Kasper, Employment and Legislative Coordinator of the American Association of Nurse Anesthetists, deserves a word of thanks for his help in supplying sample contracts and labor information.

My secretary Ann Lake is an excellent typist, excells in language usage, and was invaluable in typing and editing the manuscript.

A final word of thanks goes to family and close friends for their love and support.

Foreword

This practical legal guide for nurse anesthetists is richly illustrated and referenced with current and specific case law. The author's experiences and breadth of knowledge have been garnered through years of anesthesia practice as a clinician, educator, administrator, and student of the legal process.

The importance of this text lies in its serving several needs. It offers students and clinicians alike a basic knowledge of the historical development and current status of the American legal system. Additionally, precise and timely information is presented regarding legal topics inherent in the daily practice of anesthesia.

A thorough discussion of anesthesia practice and the law offers practical points regarding the legalities of regional anesthesia and the prevention of suits. The author's in-depth exploration of the concepts of employment and labor law also allows the examination of anesthesia cases involving legal parameters other than negligence. These unique facets, seldom if ever found in other texts, combined with the presented theory base produce a volume that has a place in the library of every professional providing anesthesia care.

Linda C. Larson, C.R.N.A., M.A.
Assistant Director/Education
Kaiser-Permanente School of Nurse Anesthesia
Los Angeles, California

1
Legal History of Nurse Anesthesia—An Introduction

> "The reason for the innovation of the nurse anesthetist was simply the very evident need for better service, which can only come from primacy of work."
> —Agatha C. Hodgins (1877–1945)
> First President of the American Association
> of Nurse Anesthetists

The origin of nurse anesthesia in the United States can be traced to the latter part of the 19th century. In 1877, Sister Mary Bernard entered St. Vincent's Hospital in Erie, Pennsylvania for training as a nurse. Within a year she was called upon to assume the duties of administering anesthesia.

Although records are scarce, evidence that nurses were trained in the administration of anesthesia in various parts of the country docs exist. Alice Magaw (1860–1925) administered anesthesia at the Mayo Clinic and reported 1042 cases of ether anesthesia in 1900. Agatha C. Hodgins was trained as an anesthetist by Dr. George C. Crile of Cleveland. Miss Hodgins was noted for her skill in administering anesthesia as well as her ability to teach both doctors and nurses her techniques.

As a profession, nurse anesthesia was intrinsically affected by both world wars.[1] The role of anesthetists in these and subsequent wars, including Korea and Vietnam, was significant. The need for trained people to adminster anesthesia accelerated with the number of wounded. Nurse anesthetists were invaluable in performing this service in military and field hospitals, while other civilian nurse anesthetists maintained the standard of care in the States.

While tradition and history strongly support the utilization of nurses in the administration of anesthesia, the challenges to the profession have been persistent. Statistics show that over 50 percent of the anesthetics given in the United States are administered by nurse anesthetists. These statistics also verify the geographic maldistribution of nurse anesthetists and anesthesiologists.[2,3]

The question that frequently arises when nurse anesthesia practice is challenged is whether or not the administration of anesthesia constitutes the practice of medicine. Nurse Practice Acts, which include definition of nurse anesthetists, along with Federal and State Health and Safety Codes provide statutory recognition of the profession (see Chapter 3).

The question of whether nurse anesthesia is an illegal practice of medicine was addressed in 1936 by the California Supreme Court in a landmark decision that has been quoted in subsequent cases; in Chalmers v. Nelson, nurse anesthesia practice was verified from a common law perspective.

Two practicing physicians and surgeons, on behalf of themselves and all other doctors, brought this injunction proceeding to restrain the defendant Nelson, a licensed and registered nurse employed by the defendant hospital, from administering general anesthetics in connection with operations. Such practice by the defendant is asserted to constitute the illegal practice of medicine, in violation of the Medical Practice Act. Judgment went for the defendants and plaintiffs appealed.

"Appellants' arguments are directed to the proposition that defendants are illegally practicing medicine. The findings, which are amply supported by the testimony in this case, show conclusively that everything which was done by the nurse, Dagmar A. Nelson, in the present instance, and by nurses generally, in the administration of anesthetics, was and is done under the immediate supervision of the operating surgeons and his assistants. Such method seems to be the the uniform practice in operating rooms. There was much testimony as to the recognized practice of permitting nurses to administer anesthetics and hypodermics. One of the plaintiff's witnesses testified to what seems to be the established and *uniformly accepted practice and procedure* followed by surgeons and nurses, and that is that it is not diagnosing nor prescribing by nurses within the meaning of the Medical Practice

Legal History of Nurse Anesthesia

Act. We are led further to accept this practice and procedure as established when we consider the evidence of the many surgeons who supported the contenton of the defendant nurse, and whose qualifications to testify concerning the practice of medicine in this community and elsewhere were established beyond doubt."

Chalmers-Francis v. Nelson, 6 Cal. 2d 402 (1936)

The Chalmers-Francis decision was quoted in another legal opinion which addressed the practice of medicine and the delegation of functions to others. The court in this case concluded:

"Under some circumstances, persons not licensed to practice medicine in California may legally perform some medical acts, including the administration of anesthesia. . . . .

"It is generally recognized that the function of nurses and physicians overlap to some extent, and a licensed nurse, when acting under the direction and supervision of a licensed physician is permitted to perform certain tasks, which without such direction and supervision, would constitute the illegal practice of medicine or surgery."

Magit v. Board of Medical Examiners, 57 C. 2d 17 Cal. Rptr. 488 (1956)

Nurse anesthesia was the first nursing specialty to seek independent recognition in education and certification. Other groups, such as nurse midwives, critical care, and operating room nurses, currently are following in the path opened up by anesthetists. This path is leading to statutory and judicial recognition of their expanded nursing functions.

Inherent in the legal recognition of a profession is accountability to the public. Lawsuits for malpractice attest to the accountability and vulnerability of the profession of nurse anesthesia and reinforce the necessity for each individual to be knowledgeable in this area and to assume responsibility for his or her professional actions.

The nurse anesthetist of the 1980s is a well-educated, clinically competent professional. Through programs established by the American Association of Nurse Anesthetists (AANA) and the respective councils on accreditation, certification, recertification, and practice, the status and public recognition of the profession will be expanded.

In this book a study of the legal status of nurse anesthetists, judical decisions and opinions affecting the practice, and trends that will influence the future are presented in a comprehensive form.

The reader may be frustrated by the paucity of facts concerning the management of an anesthetic or some of the opinions expressed by the courts in the cases reported in this book. The author recognizes these limitations, but believes the educational value outweighs the lack of information available.

REFERENCES

1. American Association of Nurse Anesthetists: A 50 Year Retrospective. Park Ridge, Illinois, AANA, 1981
2. Biggins D, Bakutis A et al: Survey of Anesthesia Service—1971. AANA J 39:5, 1971
3. Supply, Need and Distribution of Anesthesiologists and Nurse Anesthetists in the U.S.—1972 and 1980. PHS, DHEW Publications, 1976

2
American Legal System

The nurse anesthetist will find it useful to understand the sources and origins of law, recent court decisions, and legislative enactments relative to clinical practice.

Law is the aggregate of rules and principles by which society is governed. It is a dynamic field reflecting change and growth in society. Modern law is derived from four basic sources: statutes, regulations of government agencies, court decisions, and Attorney General opinions.

COMMON LAW

Common law is a system of jurisprudence inherited by the United States from England. It is a system of "judge-made" law that applies the principles of *precedent* rather than legislative enactment. The essence of common law is the fact that law by judicial precedent is as binding as law enacted by the legislature. The common law system is applied in all states except Louisiana, where the civil law code derived from French law is still followed.

The concept of precedent or *stare decisis* is utilization of rules and principles applied in a previous decision to decide the current case. A court may recognize distinctions between the precedent and the current case or may conclude that a particular common law rule is no longer in accord with the needs of society, thus departing from precedent. This is seen in medical judicial rulings where advances in medicine and communications render previous decisions obsolete.

Common law principles are summarized by Oliver Wendell Holmes:

> The life of the law has not been logic, it has been experience. The felt necessities of the time, the prevalent moral and political theories, intentions of public policy, avowed or unconscious even in the prejudice which judges share with their fellowman, have a good deal more to do than the syllogism in determining the rules by which men should be governed. The law embodies the story of a nation's development through the centuries, and it cannot be dealt with as if it contained only axions and corollaries of a book of mathematics. In order to know what it is, we must know what it has been, and what it tends to become.

Holmes, OW: The Common Law. Boston, Little, Brown & Co, 1881

CONSTITUTONS

The Constitution of the United States is the overriding legal force governing both the common law and the state statutes. It provides for a balance of powers between the legislative, judicial, and executive branches of the government by a system of checks and balances.

While each state has drafted its own constitution, no state can pass or enforce laws that transgress the mandates of the Federal Constitution. Both the United States and the state constitutions may be amended and are subject to interpretation by the Supreme Court, as dictated by changes in law, society, economics, and science.

COURT SYSTEM

The court system in the United States is divided into two separate divisions, federal and state, with each hearing cases that fall within its specific jurisdiction.

Federal

The federal court system, as established by the United States Constitution, has jurisdiction over a limited category of cases such as maritime, copyrights, violations of federal statutes, controversies between individuals and the United States government, or between various states.

The United States Supreme Court exercises appellate jurisdiction in both federal and state matters. The highest court of the land will review decisions from state supreme courts, to determine whether or not there was a violation of the United States Constitution. It will generally not review issues of state law that are not of particular importance outside the state.

The Supreme Court exercises a great deal of discretion in determining which cases it will hear and usually accepts only those cases that have application to all citizens. As the court of last resort over state and federal courts, the United States Supreme Court is the final interpreter of the Constitution.

State Laws

The court structure of the individual states is established by the state legislature and varies with individual states. Each state generally has a triple hierarchy of courts consisting of lower levels, trial, and appellate divisions. The lower level, often called municipal courts, are not courts of record and may be divided into such areas as traffic, small claims, civil, and criminal.

Trial courts of general jurisdiction may be called superior or district courts and are courts of record. Cases heard in trial courts may be appealed from the lower courts or trials *"de novo,"* new trials. Trial courts follow formal precedures, presided over by a judge and have the proceedings recorded by a court stenographer.

Decisions from lower courts may be appealed to the higher courts of the state (appellate and state supreme court). The function of the appellate courts is to decide issues of law after hearing arguments on both sides. They may determine that there was no error of law and affirm the decision of the lower court or they may reverse the decision or remand the case back for a new trial. The decisions of the appellate courts are regarded as precedent setting and are recorded in legal books.

ADVERSARY SYSTEM

The American legal system, under common law, follows what is known as "adversary" proceedings. This system provides that both sides of a controversy will be represented by legal counsel, who will present their case in the most favorable and forceful manner possible. The adversarial system permits discovery to attain facts, establish liability and responsibility, along with rights and duties. Each side, regardless of status, has the opportunity to have its case heard in a neutral forum following strict rules of evidence and procedure. The essence of the adversary system is that each side will have "its day in court" and that truth will be defined and justice realized.

ANATOMY OF A LAWSUIT

A nurse anesthetist named in a negligence suit has commented: "once you receive the notice that you have been sued, your life changes from that moment on." Lawsuits from the initial incident through exhaustion of all appeals is a structured process. The ultimate function of the legal system in a civil suit is to resolve disputes between the parties in a manner consistent with the applicable law and principles and to do so within a time frame that will make any relief granted meaningful. The typical negligence civil suit can be divided into three separate stages: preliminary (discovery), trial, and appeal.

Preliminary Stage

Starting with the actual incident and ending with the beginning of the trial, this preparatory phase is often the most critical time in a negligence lawsuit. The sequence of events starts with the filing of a document called a *complaint* by the plaintiff (patient), who contends that his or her legal rights have been infringed by the conduct of one or more persons called defendants. The complaint is filed with the court and a copy is served on the defendant. The complaint specifies the facts that the plaintiff's attorney hopes to establish and the dollar value of the harm caused by the defendant's alleged negligence.

The defendants through their attorney file a *response* or answer in which they deny all allegations in the complaint. The response

American Legal System

may contain affirmative defenses and counter claims against the plaintiff.

After all of the pleadings are properly filed, both sides begin the lengthy process of *discovery* where all the pertinent facts of the case are elicited. Methods of obtaining these facts include review of all charts and records and utilization of depositions and interrogations.

Deposition

A deposition is an oral question and answer session, under oath, where the attorneys seek to discuss what testimony and evidence will be confronting them in the lawsuit. All questions and answers are recorded verbatim and are transcribed in booklet form for use by all parties involved.

Interrogatory

Interrogatory represents another discovery mechanism and is the written equivalent of the depostion. The questions are typed and, within a prescribed period of time, the answers are prepared and filed. Interrogatories are utilized by both the plaintiff and defense attorneys to probe and identify the key points in chart entries and procedures involving the incident in question.

Expert witnesses are utilized in the discovery phase of professional negligence cases. They review charts, records, and depositions and offer an opinion regarding whether or not the defendants met the standard of care.

Settlements

Most nurse anesthetists have malpractice insurance coverage, whether through a personal policy or through coverage by their employer. Upon notification of an impending suit, the nurse anesthetist must immediately notify his or her insurer, who in turn retains an attorney to defend the case.

The defense attorney and insurance company may recommend an out of court settlement. Settlements may be determined based on the medical-legal analysis of the facts of the case, the severity of the injury, and experience and judgment of the attorney. A settlement is *not* to be considered an admission of guilt, but simply as the best way of resolving the dispute for all the parties involved.

TRIAL

The actual trial begins with the selection of the jury, and is followed by the opening statements of both sides. In these opening remarks, the attorneys outline the nature of their case, point to theories that they will be attempting to prove or disprove, and allude to the type of witnesses they will call.

Plaintiff's Case

After the opening statements, the plaintiff's case is presented. A succession of witnesses are called and exhibits are presented in an attempt to substantiate the claims against the defendant.

Defendant's Case

The defense presents evidence in support of its position. The evidence presented by the defense is not necessarily relevant to the material introduced earlier by the plaintiff. The actual defendants involved—surgeon, anesthesiologist, etc.—may be called and examined by the defense attorney. Witnesses and experts for both sides may be cross-examined by the opposing attorney.

Closing Statements

Attorneys from each side conclude by giving closing arguments to the jury and summarizing the evidence presented and what they believe the evidence proves. The judge then gives the jury instruction, explaining the legal principles they should apply to the facts of the case in order to arrive at either a plaintiff or defense verdict.

Jury

The jury deliberates, reaches a verdict, establishes how much harm, if any, the plaintiff suffered, and decides whether the defendants are liable for the harm done to the plaintiff. The jury will also

American Legal System

set a monetary damage award when a verdict for the plaintiff is rendered.

Appeal

Any of the parties to the litigation has the right to appeal their case to a higher court. The issues on appeal are somewhat different from those presented at trial, because the appellate court does not retry a case or hear all of the evidence again. They do not consider matters of fact, since they were determined at the trial court level. They will review the transcripts of the trial proceedings to determine whether rulings of legal issues were in error.

The appellate courts do not reconsider findings of fact on the premise that the judge and jury have the opportunity to see and evaluate the impressions they have made through testimony. An appellate court's application of the law as applied to the fact situation is called the *holding* of the case, thus the precedent decision.

Evidence

The rules of evidence are that part of the law that governs *how* a trial is conducted. Evidence includes the testimony of witnesses, introduction of records, documents, exhibitions, objects, and all or any other probative matter offered for the purpose of arriving at the truth and settling the dispute at trial. Admissable evidence must be truthful (have veracity), the best available, from a competent source, and relevant to the issues of the case.

The two types of evidence commonly considered are direct and circumstantial. Direct proof is normally based on the actual observation of witnesses, whereas circumstantial evidence are the secondary or indirect facts by which a principal fact may be rationally inferred.

Medical Records

The patient's hospital records will be presented as evidence in a negligence case. All information recorded on the chart will be carefully analyzed by both sides and utilized in the presentation of their cases. It is important that notations on medical records be accurate, legible, and timely as the writer may have to defend their veracity. Further discussion on anesthesia records will be found in Chapter 6 on prevention of anesthesia lawsuits.

Expert Testimony

Because juries are composed of laymen, expert testimony is valued in medical cases where the experience and expertise of the witness is offered to help base a decision on whether the conduct by the defendant was negligent. Expert testimony is permitted and encouraged in those areas where the jurors have no knowledge or expertise, such as the medical field.

An expert witness must generally be knowledgeable about the particular medical problem or technique in question. The Federal Rules of Evidence speak in broad terms of an expert qualified by "knowledge, skills, experience, or education. . . ." Fed. R. Evid. 702

In litigation involving nurse anesthetists, anesthesiologists are predominately used as expert witnesses. There does appear to be a recent trend in more nurse anesthetists fulfilling this essential function in malpractice proceedings. Hopefully, this trend will continue so that members of the same profession will give expert testimony as to the standards of care of that profession.

ARBITRATION

Arbitration is a method of settling legal disputes without litigation. If two parties submit to arbitration, the decision of the arbitrator is final, subject only to a limited right of appeal to the courts, and the parties are barred from litigating the same claim at a later date in court.

3
Statutory and Regulatory Law

The body of laws known as statutes has an impact on nurse anesthetist practice in the form of nurse practice acts, medical practice acts, health and safety codes, and a variety of rules, regulations, legal opinions, and judicial interpretations. From a historic perspective, the federal government has been committed to support and safeguard health for more that 80 years. Early laws simply stated minimal educational standards with little, if any, control over the practice itself.

Statutory laws regulating nursing, medicine, and health care practice are primarily defined and enforced on an individual state basis. All states have laws that define professional practice along with education and licensure requirements for the particular profession.

A *regulation* is a law that has been adopted by a state regulatory agency such as the Board of Registered Nursing. State regulatory agencies are given power and authority by legislatures to make the statutes workable. Regulations have the same legal impact as statutes.

The Attorney General, as the chief lawyer of the state, is often called upon to issue written opinions and interpretations of laws and regulations. These opinions are treated by state agencies virtually the same as statutes, regulations, or court decisions. An example of an Attorney General opinion that affects Certified Registered Nurse Anesthetist (C.R.N.A.) practice on regional anesthesia in the state of California will be discussed later.

NURSE PRACTICE ACTS

Nurse anesthetists practice under the sphere of the Nurse Practice Act and the rules and regulations established by the nursing board of the individual state. Recent trends show that nurse anesthetists have achieved legal recognition in nurse practice acts along with other nursing specialty groups such as nurse midwifes, nurse practitioners, pediatric, and psychiatric nurse clinicians.

The recognition of specialty nursing groups differs from state to state, but generally educational and certification requirements for the groups are defined as well as the scope of practice. It is imperative that each C.R.N.A. be aware of the licensure requirements in the particular state of employment. The old adage, "ignorance of the law is no excuse," is easily applied to this area. One must know the exact legal framework of the nursing laws, along with the rules and regulations that further delineate the manner in which the law will be enforced.

Table 3-1 shows extracts from various Nurse Practice Acts that recognize nurse anesthetists. These samples are sections taken directly from the acts and are by no means complete. The reader should refer to the entire law of the state which can be obtained from the Board of Registered Nurses in the state capital.

Table 3-1
Extracts from Nurse Practice Acts

Alabama
  Section VI. Expanded roles
    1. C.R.N.A.
      1.2. *Functions*
        a. Administers anesthetics and ancillary services under the direction or supervision of a duly licensed physician or dentist.
        b. Applies the nursing process to the patient by assessment, intervention, and evaluation as this process pertains to the practice of anesthesia.

Arkansas
  Part III. Rules and regulations
    Section 1. Accountability

Statutory and Regulatory Law

The nurse practicing in the expanded role is individually responsible and accountable for her practice.

Section 2. Collaboration with a licensed physician

The nurse practicing in the expanded role of C.R.N.A. shall function in collaboration with physicians or dentists in accordance with Sec. 3, Act 613 passed 1979, Act 14 passed 1980, and of these regulations. She will conduct her practice consistently with the guidelines and scope of practice described in Sec. 3 and Part 4, Secs. 1,2, and 3 below.

Section 3. Guidelines

Every nurse practicing in the expanded role of C.R.N.A. shall practice in accordance with written guidelines developed in collaboration with a licensed physician or with the appropriate medical staff of the institution employing the nurse and in compliance with the Statutes of the State of Arkansas. These guidelines shall include established procedures for the handling of common medical problems in the practice setting and specialty area of the nurse. They shall include the scope of practice as defined below for the specialty area of the nurse. They shall specifically address the degree to which supervision, collaboration, and independent action is required for actions of the nurse, including when such actions involve medical determination to administer a particular treatment to a patient. Guidelines shall provide for the performance by the nurse of acts including, but not limited to, evaluation, diagnosis, and treatment. These guidelines shall be reviewed jointly at least annually, and revised when necessary.

Part IV. Scope of practice for categories of nurses practicing in the expanded role of C.R.N.A.

Section 1. Nurse anesthetist

C.R.N.A.s shall be authorized to administer anesthesia. Their performance shall be under the overall direction of the director of anesthesia services or his or her qualified anesthetist designees; otherwise their performance shall be under the overall direction of the physician responsible for the patient's care.

Section 2. The extent of services, responsibilities, and required supervision of nurse anesthetists; and the accompanying responsibilities of attending physicians must be defined by each hospital or clinic in a policy statement, job description, protocol, or other appropriate document.

Table 3-1 (continued)
Florida
Chapter 464. Nursing
(a) The nurse anesthetist may, to the extent authorized by established protocol approved by the medical staff of the facility in which the anesthetic service is performed, perform, in addition to the general functions in subsection (3), any or all of the following:
   1. Determine the health status of the patient as it relates to the risk factors and to the anesthetic management of the patient through the performance of the general functions.
   2. Based on history, physical assessment, and supplemental laboratory results, determine with the consent of the responsible physician, the appropriate type of anesthesia within the framework of protocol.
   3. Order, under protocol, preanesthetic medication.
   4. Perform, under protocol, procedures commonly used to render the patient insensible to pain during the performance of surgical, obstetric, therapeutic, or diagnostic clinical procedures. This shall include ordering and administering regional, spinal, and general anesthesia, inhalation agents and techniques, intravenous agents, and techniques of hypnosis.
   5. Order and/or perform monitoring procedures indicated as pertinent to the anesthetic health care management of the patient.
   6. Support life functions during anesthesia health care, including induction and intubation procedures, the use of appropriate mechanical supportive devices, and the management of fluid, electrolyte, and blood component balances.
   7. Recognize and take appropriate corrective action for abnormal patient responses to anesthesia, adjunctive medication, or other forms of therapy.
   8. Recognize and treat cardiac arrythmias while patient is under anesthetic care.
   9. Participate in management of the patient while in postanesthesia recovery area, including ordering the administration of fluids and drugs. Place special peripheral and central venous and arterial lines for blood sampling and monitoring as appropriate.

Georgia
Chapter 84–10A. C.R.N.A.
84–1002a. When anesthesia may be administered by a C.R.N.A.:
In any case where it is lawful for a duly licensed physician practicing medicine under the laws of this State to administer anesthesia, such anesthesia may also lawfully be administered by a C.R.N.A. provided that such anesthesia is administered under the direction and responsibility of a duly licensed physician with training or experience in anesthesia.

Statutory and Regulatory Law

Kansas

60-10-14. Function of the advanced registered nurse practitioner in the expanded role of C.R.N.A.

An advanced registered nurse practitioner functioning in the expanded role of certified nurse anesthetist performs in an interdependent role as a member of a physician- or dentist-directed health care team. The certified registered anesthetist shall:

(a) Conduct of pre- and postanesthesia visit and assessment with appropriate documentation.

(b) Develop an anesthesia care plan with the physician or dentist which includes medications and anesthetic agents.

(c) Induce and maintain anesthesia at the required levels.

(d) Support life functions during the perioperative period.

(e) Recognize and take appropriate action for untoward patient responses during anesthesia.

(f) Provide professional observation and management of patient's emergence from anesthesia.

(g) Participate in life support of the patient for whatever cause.

Maryland

.02. C.R.N.A.—standards of practice

A. A nurse anesthetist certified under these regulations may engage in the practice of nurse anesthesia as that term is defined in Regulation .01A, above.

B. A nurse anesthetist certified under these regulations shall collaborate with an anesthesiologist, licensed physician, or dentist in the following manner:

(1) An anesthesiologist, licensed physician, or dentist shall be physically available to the nurse anesthetist for consultation at all times during the administration of and recovery from anesthesia.

(2) An anesthesiologsit shall be available for consultation to the nurse anesthetist for other aspects of the practice of nurse anesthesia. If an anesthesiologist is not available, a licensed physician or dentist shall be available to provide this type of consultation.

C. A C.R.N.A. shall report to the Board [of Nursing] the name of the collaborating anesthesiologist, physician, or dentist. When the Board receives the name of the collaborating anesthesiologist, licensed physician, or dentist, this information shall be forwarded to the appropriate Regulatory Board.

D. A C.R.N.A. has the right and the obligation to refuse to perform any delegated act, whether oral or written if, in the C.R.N.A.s judgment, it is an unsafe or invalidly prescribed medical act.

Table 3-1 (continued)

Massachusetts

244 CMR. Board of registration of nursing

(4) Nurse Anesthetist. The area of practice of a nurse anesthetist is the preparation of a patient for anesthesia, its administration, and the provision of postoperative care according to guidelines approved and developed in compliance with section 4.22 and which satisfy the requirements of section 4.24 and are more precisely delineated in the separate paragraphs contained in the subdivisions below.

(a) Performing an immediate preoperative patient evaluation

(b) Selecting an anesthetic agent

(c) Including and maintaining anesthesia and managing intraoperative pain relief

(d) Supporting life functions during the induction and period of anesthesia, including intratracheal intubation, monitoring of blood loss and replacement and electrolytes, and the maintenance of cardiovascular and respiratory function

(e) Recognizing abnormal patient responses to anesthesia, any adjunctive medication, or other form of therapy and taking corrective action

(f) Providing professional observation and resuscitative care during the immediate postoperative period and until a patient has regained control of his vital functions

(g) Such other additional professional activities as authorized by the guidelines under which a particular nurse anesthetist practices

Nevada

632.010. Definition of words and terms as used in this chapter

3. Certified registered nurse anesthetist means a person who has completed a nationally accredited program in the science of anesthesia, who, when licensed as a registered nurse under the provisions of this chapter, administers anesthetic agents to individuals under the care of those persons licensed by the State of Nevada to practice dentistry, surgery, or obstetrics.

New Hampshire

5. Administration of anesthesia

A currently licensed registered nurse may legally administer anesthetics under the following conditions:

a. has completed a program for nurse anesthetists accredited by the AANA;

b. is certified as a registered nurse anesthetist; and

Statutory and Regulatory Law

    c. administers such anesthesia under the direction of and in the presence of a licensed physician or dentist. Note: "In the presence" means in the same room, an adjoining room, or within the same surgial or obstetric suite.

New Jersey

IV. Delivery of the anesthesia service by the certified nurse anesthetist
The C.R.N.A. shall provide but is not limited to:
- (a) Conduct a preanesthesia evaluation in consultation with the responsible physician which shall include a review of previous anesthesia history, history and physical assessment, laboratory values, and other pertinent data regarding patient status.
- (b) Render the patient insensible to pain during the performance of surgical, obstetric, dental, diagnostic, and therapeutic procedures. The aforesaid shall include the selection and utilization of the following techniques: inhalation, regional, intravascular, rectal, oral, subcutaneous, intramuscular, intraperitoneal, and hypnosis.
- (c) Perform monitoring procedures indicated as pertinent to the anesthesia health care management of the patient.
- (d) Support life functions during anesthesia health care by utilizing induction and intubation procedures, using appropriate mechanical supportive devices, managing fluid, electrolyte, and blood component balances, and administering drugs as necessary.
- (e) Recognize and institute corrective action for abnormal patient responses to anesthesia, adjunctive medication, and other forms of therapy and document same.
- (f) Participate in the management of the patient while in the postanesthesia recovery room.
- (g) Place peripheral, central venous, and arterial lines for blood sampling and monitoring as appropriate.
- (h) Conduct a postanesthesia evaluation which includes assessment of patient response to the anesthesia management.
- (i) Function as an active member of the life support team.

New Mexico

67.2–4.1. Administration of general anesthesia—exceptions
It shall be unlawful for any person, other than a person licensed in New Mexico to practice medicine, osteopathy, or dentistry, or a C.R.N.A. when acting under the direction of and in the immediate area of a licensed physician or dentist, to administer general anesthesia to any person. Nothing in this section prohibits a person licensed in the healing arts from administering local anesthesia or from using hypnosis.

Table 3-1 (continued)

Oklahoma
567.51. C.R.N.A.
3. Administers anesthesia under the supervision of and in the immediate presence of a physician licensed to practice medicine, an osteopath, or a dentist; is hereby recognized to administer anesthesia for any physician licensed to practice medicine in the State of Oklahoma or for an osteopath or dentist licensed in the State of Oklahoma and shall have the right to use both the title "Certified Registered Nurse Anesthetist" and the abbreviation "C.R.N.A."

South Carolina
Chapter 91.
(f) A professional nurse may perform additional acts requiring special education and training which are recognized jointly by the medical and nursing professions as proper for such nurse to perform if licensed under this chapter and recognized by the Board of Nursing through its rules and regulations.

South Dakota
H B 1260 Section 2.
(3) A C.R.N.A. in this State shall be required to submit evidence to the Board [of Nursing] that she is qualified to so practice, and shall be licensed or certified as provided in this chapter.
Section 3.
A C.R.N.A., in addition to performing all those functions within the scope of practice of a registered nurse as provided in chapter 39–9, may accept the delegation of and perform the following medical functions:
  (1) Develop an anesthesia care plan
  (2) Induce anesthesia
  (3) Maintain anesthesia at the required levels
  (4) Support life functions during the perioperative period
  (5) Recognize and take appropriate action for untoward patient responses during anesthesia
  (6) Provide professional observation and management of the patient's emergence from anesthesia during the immediate postoperative period
  (7) Conduct postanesthesia visit and assessment when appropriate
  (8) Participate in the life support of the patient for whatever cause
The medical functions shall be performed only under the supervision of a licensed physician responsible for the medical care of the patient.

Utah
58.31.91. Advanced or special categories of licensure
Registered nurses with advanced or specialized preparations who meet the criteria set forth in the rules and regulations and pay any additional

Statutory and Regulatory Law

fees provided for application for special licensure, shall have their professional nursing license designate their advanced or special category of practice including, but not limited to:
  (1) Nurse practitioners
  (2) Nurse anesthetists
  (3) Nurse specialists

Virginia
XII. Related regulations
  1. A nurse who has completed a nurse anesthetist practitioner program accredited by the AANA may practive under the direct supervision of a licensed physician including a licensed podiatrist or dentist pending receipt of the results of the first certification examination for which he or she is eligible.

Washington
V. Brief overview of C.R.N. practice
C.R.N. Anesthesia
The C.R.N. in anesthesia practice provides nursing and anesthesia services to persons of any age group requiring a combination of these services. This C.R.N. manages life support functions under the stress of anesthetic and surgical procedures.

The C.R.N. in anesthesia practice with prescriptive authority may prescribe a variety of legend drugs, mainly those involved in life support, pain relief, cardiac and respiratory problems, and fluid, electrolyte, and metabolic disturbances.

SUSPENSION AND REVOCATION OF LICENSE

Boards of registered nurses have the authority to suspend or revoke the license of a person found in violation of specific norms of conduct. Such violations may include obtaining the license by fraud, unprofessional or illegal conduct, or performance of specific actions prohibited by the board. Procedures by which the board carries out formal suspension or revocation are usually specified in the licensing law or in the rules and regulations of the board. These administrative proceedings offer the nurse due process through the following mechanisms: (1) notification of the charges; and (2) formal hearing where the nurse may present a defense and be represented by legal counsel.

Since the hearing by the nursing boards are administrative in nature, most states authorize judicial review of board proceedings.

The following cases illustrate higher court rulings on state board decisions.

Ms. Tighe, while employed as a private duty nurse at Arlington Memorial Hospital, on three dates was charged with tampering with tubexes prefilled with the narcotic Demerol® [meperidine hydrochloride]. At the hearing conducted by the State Board of Nurse Examiners, the Commonwealth produced evidence tending to show that Nurse Tighe signed for tubexes of Demerol® for administration to her patient. Some of the tubexes she returned as unused or as inadvertently spoiled. It was determined later that the tubexes were emptied of their contents of Demerol® and refilled with saline solution. There was also evidence that she altered records concerning her administration of Demerol® to a patient.

The board suspended her license for 1 year.

On appeal, Pennsylvania Commonwealth Court ruled that the State Board of Nurse Examiners acted properly. The court stated that the 1-year suspension was not unappropriately harsh in view of her fraudulent and deceitful acts.

Tighe v. Commonwealth of Pennsylvania, State Board of Nurse Examiners, 397 A. 2d 1261 Commonwealth Ct. of Pa. (1979)

An important case involving a nurse anesthetist and his interpretation of the state board rule on the administration of anesthesia is found in recent Pennsylvania law in McCarl v. Commonwealth of Pennsylvania State Board of Nurse Examiners.

The regulation in the Pennsylvania code at issue states that:

"The administration of anesthesia is a proper function of a registered nurse and is a function regulated by this section; such function shall not be performed unless all of the following provisions are met: (1) The registered nurse has successfully completed the educational program of a school of nurse anesthetists accredited by the AANA. (2) The registered nurse is certified as a Registered Nurse Anesthetist by the AANA within 1 year following completion of the educational program. (3) The registered nurse administers such anesthesia under the direction of and in the presence of a licensed physician or dentist."

The facts recorded in the court ruling are sparse, but indicate a differing opinion by the surgeon and anesthesiologist as to the meaning, under the regulation, of *administering* of anesthesia and the meaning of "under the direction" of a physician or dentist.

The nurse anesthetist apparently induced anesthesia by needle without the supervising anesthesiologist being present, although the surgeon was physically present in the operating room. The Board of Nurse Examiners

Statutory and Regulatory Law

ordered a formal reprimand against the nurse anesthetist for *"willfuly* violating" one of the regulations.

The nurse anesthetist appealed the Board ruling and argued that (1) the finding of the willful violation of a regulation of the Board was not supported by substantial evidence; (2) that the Board may only *suspend* or *revoke* a license, but is without authority to *formally reprimand* for a violation; and (3) that he was denied due process of the law during the Board proceedings.

The Pennsylvania Commonwealth Court upheld the Board's reprimand. They said: "The record clearly supports the Board's determination that appellant willfuly violated a regulation of the Board. It established that appellant was aware of his responsibility to secure the presence of a directing physician; that he knew that the physician whom he ought to have present was not, in fact, present during the administration of the anesthetic, and that appellant was aware that the physician who was present did not know that he was about to administer the anesthetic."

In footnoting their opinion, the court also said: "It is significant that even though appellant admitted that this physician was not present, appellant nevertheless noted in the anesthesia record, in his own handwriting, that the physician *was* present and supervising.

"The physician's (surgeon's) deposition . . . makes it abundantly clear that the appellant made no effort to make the physician aware of what was happening, that the physician had absolutely no inkling of what was happening, and that the physician, in fact, had his back to the appellant when the anesthesia was administered."

Regarding the second argument that the Board may suspend or revoke a license, but not reprimand the licensee, the court said: "The Board found that a violation had occurred. Clearly then it could have revoked or suspended appellant's license. It chose, nevertheless, to be lenient and impose a formal reprimand—a sanction not specifically referred to in the law. Given the power to suspend or revoke, certainly the Board had authority to invoke the lesser penalty."

The court, on the appellant's contention of denial of due process, found the argument to be without merit and affirmed the Board's ruling of a reprimand.

Although the majority ruling of a court is what becomes binding, legal scholars recognize that very good law is often written by the minority or dissenting judges. The dissent in McCarl written by Judge Craig probably presents a more realistic analysis of the facts. Judge Craig wrote:

"I must respectfully dissent on the ground that the record does not establish that the appellant nurse 'willfuly violated' the regulation. . . . The records shows that the surgeon witness and anesthesiologist witness held different opinions as to the meaning, under the regulation, of *administration* of anesthesia and the meaning of *under the direction* of a physician or dentist. It is undisputed that a physician was present in the operating room at all times material to appellant's actions. It is also undisputed that Dr. Carter, appellant's anesthesiologist supervisor, was present in the operating room part of the time.

"Because Dr. Carter was not present when appellant initially induced the anesthesia by needle, and because the physician present at that time was not his supervisor and was not paying attention, appellant has been deemed guilty of a willful violation. However, one of the problems causing dispute among the expert medical witnesses is the ambiguity of the term 'adminiisters' in the regulation with reference to the administration of anesthesia. Does it refer only to the initial induction of anesthesia, or does it refer to the entire procedure from beginning to end, during part of which appellant's physician/supervisor was present? The adjudication of the Board is clearly confused on this point, sometimes using the term to refer to the initial injection and, in other places, using broader meaning, as indicated by discussion of the 'commencement of administration' of anesthesia.

"With the Board itself thus approving the broader meaning, it can be seen that appellant was not guilty of any egregious falsehood when he noted 'Dr. Carter present and supervising' in the anesthesia record; that statement was true during part of the administration of anesthesia, although not throughout the entire procedure.

"The major confusion is over what it means to have the 'direction' as well as the 'presence' of a licensed physician or dentist. The parties appeared to agree that supervision by an anesthesiologist is not necessary, particularly because the hospital has more operating rooms that anesthesiologists, indicating that the supervision of an anesthesia by a physician other than an anesthesiologist would not be unusual.

"There appears to be no insistence by the Board or by the majority of this Court, that the urology resident physician, who was present, was unqualified. Although being present, he could have responded to any emergency, the burden of his inattention at the time of inducing anesthesia has been placed upon the appellant. I do not believe that appellant's failure to summon the resident physician to immediate involvement amounts to a willful violation.

"Noting that the complaint here was filed by the surgeon, it appears that the appellant nurse was caught between the differing (albeit well-meaning) viewpoints of the surgical department and the anesthesiology department, over the question of whether the regulation should be given a strict or liberal interpretation. The Board, by holding the penalty to a reprimand has indicated some awareness of the difficulties faced by the appellant.

Statutory and Regulatory Law

"If the regulation is so unclear that experienced physicians cannot agree on its meaning, the appellant's adoption of one of the interpretations should not constitute a willful violation. The decision of the Board should be reversed. In any event, it is hoped that the Board will use its good offices to clarify the meaning of this ambiguous regulation for the guidance of anesthetists hereafter."

McCarl v. Commonwealth of Pennsylvania State Board of Nurse Examiners, 39 Commonwealth Court 628 Pa. (1979)

The McCarl decision points out how a law or regulation can be interpreted differently by any number of parties involved. Nurse anesthetist McCarl and his supervising anesthesiologist interpreted the regulation quite differently than the surgeon. The Board of Registered Nurse Anesthetists and the Pennsylvania Superior Court by issuing and upholding the reprimand have presented a narrow and probably unrealistic viewpoint of supervision and direction by a physician.

MEDICAL PRACTICE ACTS

Every state clearly defines the components of medical practice through medical practice acts which permit only those individuals who meet the necessary qualifications to use the Medical Doctor (M.D.) title and to practice medicine.

Traditionally, the practice of medicine includes the three functions of diagnosis, prescription, and treatment. Although medical personnel other than a physician may actually carry out medical techniques, the physician's authority to make necessary medical judgments is in no way impaired.

Most medical practice acts provide criminal, civil, and administrative sanctions including fines, imprisonment, injunctions, and revocation of license for the unlicensed practice of medicine and for aiding and abetting another in such practice.

HEALTH AND SAFETY CODES

State laws have been enacted to regulate hospitals and other health facilities. The purpose of these laws is to license hospitals, permitting them to perform the services included within the scope of the regulation. A number of state health and safety codes are similar to the voluntary regulations of the Joint Commission on Accreditation of Hospitals (JCAH), which will be discussed in the next section.

State licensing agencies have, under constitutional police power, the duty to protect the health and safety of the citizens. For that reason, major violations of the hospital code regulations may force revocation of the license whereby patients may not be admitted. Lesser infractions may warrant a probation period or provisional licensure.

VOLUNTARY REGULATIONS

The JCAH represents a voluntary organization whose stated purpose is to establish standards for the operation of hospitals and other health related facilities and services (JCAH, Accreditation Manual for Hospitals, Chicago, 1981). Standards developed by JCAH are used in conjunction with inspection surveys to evaluate hospitals applying for accreditation.

Although hospital accreditation or re-accreditation is voluntary, there are various incentives for hospitals to seek full accreditation status. Included in these are eligibility for participation in the Medicare Program and in approved residency programs, both of which recognize JCAH accreditation. A third incentive has been the substantially lower premiums offered to accredited institutions by some liability insurance carriers.

LEGAL IMPACT OF VOLUNTARY STANDARDS

Standards drafted by the JCAH and other voluntary organizations such as the National Fire Prevention Association (NFPA) have no legal force per se. But, in certain states, these voluntary standards have been adopted as law and may be viewed as having legal force.

When courts are faced with establishing a standard of care in a malpractice action, they may apply legislative enactments.

Statutory and Regulatory Law

Section 286 of the Restatement of Torts states that "The court may adopt as the standard of conduct of a reasonable man the requirements of a legislative enactment or an administrative regulation whose purpose is found to be exclusively or in part to protect (1) a class or persons that includes the one whose interest is invaded; (2) the particular interest that is invaded; (3) that interest against the kind of harm that has resulted; and (4) that interest against the particular hazard from which the harm results." (Restatement [Second] of Torts 286 [1965])

In states where JCAH regulations are voluntary and not included in statutes, courts may allow the standards admitted as evidence to aid the jury, but they are not conclusive as standard of care.

Anesthesia services are listed in the JCAH accreditation manual. The standards in 1981 are as follows:

1. Anesthesia services shall be organized, directed, and integrated with other related services or departments of the hospital.
2. Staffing for the delivery of anesthesia care shall be related to the scope and complexity of services offered.
3. Precautions shall be taken to assure the safe administration of anesthetic agents.
4. There shall be written "policies" relating to the delivery of anesthesia care.

Nurse anesthetists should be aware of their hospital's compliance with JCAH standards and the legal impact of voluntary versus mandatory standards within the laws of their particular state.

GOOD SAMARITAN STATUTES

Most states have enacted laws called "good samaritan" statutes that relieve licensed health care professionals from liability when rendering care in an emergency situation. There is no legal duty for a licensed professional to render assistance at the scene of an emergency. The laws have been made to encourage such care without fear of civil liability.

The scope of good samaritan immunity varies from state to

state in reference to persons protected, the standard of care required, and the circumstances providing protection. An example of such a law covering registered nurses is found in the California Business and Professions Code, section 2727.5, which states: "A person licensed under this chapter who in good faith renders emergency care at the scene of an emergency which occurs outside both the place and course of his or her employment shall not be liable for any civil damages as the result of acts or omissions by such person in rendering the emergency care." This section does not grant immunity from civil damages when the person is grossly negligent.

Scope of Immunity

Under most statutes, immunity is granted only when rendering emergency care. An emergency generally is considered to be an unforeseen occurrence or combination of circumstances which call for immediate action to avoid impending danger. To be covered under the laws, care given at the scene of an emergency must be rendered outside the place and course of employment. In some jurisdictions, new laws are being enacted to extend the good samaritan laws to include nurses who are part of a hospital rescue team.

An example of this, in the California Health and Safety Code, Section 1317 reads:

". . . No act or omission of any rescue team established by any health care facility licensed under this chapter . . . done or omitted while attempting to resuscitate any person who is in danger of loss of life shall impose any liability upon the health facility, the officers, members of the staff, nurses, or employees of the health facility, including, but not limited to the members of the rescue team . . . if good faith is exercised."

"Rescue team" as used in this section, means a special group of physicians, surgeons, nurses, employees of a health facility who have been trained in cardiopulmonary resuscitation and have been designated by the health facility to attempt, in cases of emergency, to resuscitate persons who are in immediate danger of loss of life.

Good samaritan immunity does not protect health care professionals from *gross negligence,* which is defined as to exercise so slight a degree of care as to justify the belief that the person is indifferent to the interests and welfare of others.

Statutory and Regulatory Law

ATTORNEY GENERAL OPINIONS

The Attorney General of a state is often called upon to issue written opinions to questions submitted by public officials. Although these opinions are the official statements of an executive officer, issued in accordance with his authority, they are merely advisory statements and are not mandatory orders. The opinions are strongly persuasive, however, and are generally followed by executive officers and also have a significant influence on the courts in their deliberations. The opinions, as a general rule, relate to interpretations of statutes or general legal problems.

A leading Attorney General opinion that has a significant legal impact on nurse anesthesia practice is found in Calfiornia. In 1972, a state assemblyman requested an opinion from the Attorney General's Office on the following questions:

1. May nurse anesthetists administer spinal, epidural, and regional anesthesia and analgesia?
2. Who may or must supervise a nurse anesthetis, i.e., physician, dentist, osteopath, podiatrist, other nurse, etc.?
3. May nurse anesthetists administer anesthetics on a freelance basis and bill for their services?
4. What may licensed registered nurses enrolled in an approved school for anesthesiology do?

The conclusions were:

1. Registered nurses may not administer spinal, epidural, and regional anesthesia and analgesia.
2. Only physicians and surgeons licensed with the Board of Medical Examiners or the Board of Osteopathic Examiners and dentists licensed with the Board of Dental Examiners may supervise registered nurses in the administration of general anesthetics. Podiatrists licensed by the Board of Medical Examiners may not supervise registered nurses in the administration of a local anesthetic.
3. Registered nurses may administer anesthetics on a free-lance basis under the supervision of any one or more of the classes of licentiates referred to above and bill the patient for their services.
4. Licensed registered nurses enrolled in an approved school for

anesthesia may only administer general anesthesia and only if they are directed and supervised by an authorized licentiate of the healing arts.

56 Cal. Ops. Atty Gen 1 (1972)

Because of the above opinion, nurse anesthetists practicing in California do not have good legal authority for the administration of regional anesthesia.

SELECTED READING

Anderson R: Legal Boundaries of California Nursing Practice, ed 2. Sacramento, Anderson Publishing, 1981

Bertolet M, Goldsmith L: Hospital Liability: Law and Factors. New York, Practicing Law Institute, 1980

Bliss A, Cohen E: The New Health Performance. Germantown, Maryland, Aspen Systems, 1977

Dornette, WL: The legal impact of voluntary standards in civil actions against the health care provider. New York Law School Review 22:925–942, 1976–1977

Joint Commission on Accreditation of Hospitals: Accreditation Manual for Hospitals, Chicago, 1981

4
The Law of Consent

It is an inherent right for the individual to prevent unauthorized interference with his physical integrity. This right, vigorously guarded in the courts, was applied to the medical field by Justice Cardozo in 1914 when he wrote: "Every human being of adult years and sound mind has a right to determine what shall be done with his body, and a surgeon who performs an operation without his patient's consent commits . . . (a battery) for which he is liable in damages."[1] The law of consent can be divided into two categories that relate to anesthesia practice. They are consent or authorization for surgery and anesthesia and the emerging legal concept of informed consent.

CONSENT FOR SURGERY AND ANESTHESIA

Consent for surgery and anesthesia is a defense for the intentional tort of assault and battery.

Assault

Assault is defined as the intentional unlawful offer or attempt to injure another with apparent present ability to effectuate the attempt under the circumstances creating a fear of imminent peril.

Battery

The willful touching of another, whether directly or by means of a thing put in motion by the aggressor is called battery. In the medical perspective, performing surgery or administering anesthesia without the patient's consent constitutes a battery.

FORMS OF CONSENT

A patient can give consent to treatment in a number of ways.

Express

A consent given in writing by the patient is considered express consent. Such a written authorization is usually made on a standard form stating the procedure and is signed and dated by the patient. The signature should be witnessed as a method of authentication. Express written consent should be as specific as possible regarding the anticipated procedure. Written consent is usually required when the proposed diagnostic or therapeutic procedure carries some risk or danger to the patient or when the patient's body is to be invaded.[2] The written consent, properly executed and signed by the patient, is useful evidence in any subsequent legal action and should be made part of the patient's permanent record.

Implied in Fact

When a patient knowingly accepts treatment, such as rolling up his sleeve for an injection, there is said to be implied consent.

Implied in Law

The law implies consent in an emergency situation when a patient is unconscious or is otherwise unable to give consent. It is assumed that the patient would have given consent, if able. Such emergencies must generally endanger the life or health of the patient and require immediate medical intervention.

WHO MAY CONSENT

Adult

An adult who is competent may give his or her own consent. For these purposes, competency is defined as an ability to understand the nature and consequences of that to which one is asked to consent.[3] Consent of the person requiring treatment must be obtained. The spouse of the patient lacks legal capacity to give consent for the patient unless the spouse has been declared legal guardian or conservator.

Minors

Parents or legal guardians may give consent for their children. In many states, minor children who meet certain qualifications may sign for their own medical treatment. In California, for example, minors under 18 have the legal capacity to consent to medical treatment if they are living away from home and managing their own financial affairs, on active duty with armed forces, or married. Those under 18 in California may also consent to specific procedures relating to pregnancy, abortion, reportable diseases, rape, and sexual assault.[4]

WITHDRAWAL OF CONSENT

The laws relating to consent are determined by statute in each state. Anesthetists are advised to check with hospital administrators as to the particular laws in their respective states.

A legal case that illustrates a judicial interpretation of withdrawal of consent is found in Virginia.

The patient, a 44-year-old registered nurse underwent an exploratory laporotomy and oophorectomy. During the surgery, the ureter connected to her only functioning kidney was injured and the patient suffered severe postoperative complications. The patient filed suit, charging negligence and battery.

The jury found that the gynecologist had not been negligent in performing the operation and entered a verdict in his favor on the negligence count.

With respect to the battery count, the patient testified that she wanted another physician, a surgeon, present during the surgery. She testified that she made this clear to the gynecologist and that she had confirmed with the surgeon's office personnel that he would be available. On the morning of the surgery, the patient asked where the surgeon was and stated that she "did not want to be put to sleep" until he arrived. The anesthetist administered the anesthetic and the gynecologist proceeded with the surgery.

The jury found that the patient revoked her consent to surgery and awarded the patient $75,000 for battery. The gynecologist appealed.

The Virginia Supreme Court said that the relationship between the physician and patient is a consensual one. Therefore, surgery is technically a battery unless the patient or patient's authorized representative consents to it. Consent to an operation may be withdrawn and, if done timely and unequivocably, will subject the surgeon to liability for battery if the operation is continued.

Pugsley v. Privette, 263 S.E. 2d 69 (VA Sup Ct. 1980)

INFORMED CONSENT

The doctrine of informed consent dictates that the patient must receive sufficient information regarding the contemplated medical procedure so that a decision will be made with sufficient knowledge as to risks, complications, and alternatives.

Most recent legal cases where lack of informed consent was a cause of action have been decided under a negligence action instead of battery. In a leading case on informed consent, Cobbs v. Grant, the court said that when the patient consented to the procedure and an undisclosed risk developed, the occurrence of which was not an integral part or certain result of the procedure, but merely a known risk, liability would be based on negligence principles.[5]

The law of informed consent is often confusing to health care professionals because legal decisions modify earlier ones on a regular basis. Courts generally agree that certain elements of informed consent must be present for the consent to be upheld. Rulings generally have held that the patient has the right to be informed by the physician of (1) the nature of the treatment, (2) the risks, complications, and expected benefits or effects of such treatment, and (3) alternative forms of treatment.

Many courts also have held that the physician need not disclose the risks of the procedure if they are commonly considered remote and the procedure itself is simple. The risks also need not be disclosed if the patient specifically says he does not want to be informed of them or if, in the professional judgment of the physician, the disclosure of that information is not in the best interests of the patient.
From Hemelt M, Mackert M: Dynamics of Law in Nursing and Health Care. Reston Publishing Co, 1978, p 96–97. Reprinted with permission.

The rulings on this doctrine clearly state that it is the duty of a *physician* to obtain the informed consent. Because of this, nurse anesthetists are placed in the awkward position of relying on the physician to obtain proper informed consent for anesthesia. It is advisable for the person administering the anesthetic, on a preanesthetic visit, to inform the patient of the choice of agents and techniques and the possible complications and risks along with any reasonable alternatives. It is essential that a notation of informed consent be made on the patient's chart indicating what information was given to the patient and that the patient agreed.

The following legal cases illustrate judicial interpretation of the need for informed consent.

The patient, Mrs. Gravis, complained of abdominal pain and was admitted to the hospital for observation. An exploratory operation was agreed on. The surgeon obtained written consent from the patient's husband for both the operation and administration of anesthesia. In an operation under spinal anesthesia, an intestinal obstruction was found and corrected. After the operation, the patient allegedly suffered from phlebitis, bladder trouble, and partial paralysis.

The patient alleged she had never been advised that surgery was necessary and that the use of an anesthetic had not been discussed with her. She indicated that she had previously had two spinal anesthetics, and claimed that for that reason she would have not allowed a spinal anesthetic to be given to her. Both the surgeon and the anesthesiologists claimed they talked to her 2 hours before the surgery at a time when she was in possession of all her mental faculties and capable of giving consent.

The court ruled that since no emergency existed, the patient's consent should have been obtained. The record failed to establish circumstances that would have justified an operation without the patient's consent. There was no contention that the patient's spouse was authorized to consent on her behalf. The husband-wife relationship does not in itself make one spouse the agent for the other.
Gravis v. Physicians and Surgeons Hospital of Alice, 415 S.W. 2d 647 Texas (1967)

The patient's right hand was severely lacerated by the fan of his car. The orthopedic surgeon advised surgery and the patient consented to a brachial block anesthetic, which was administered by the anesthesiologist. During the process, the anesthesiologist punctured the patients right lung causing a pneumothorax.

In a malpractice suite against the orthopedic surgeon, the anesthesiologist, and the hospital, the patient claimed that the physicians failed to warn him of the complications of a brachial block and all three defendants failed to provide proper postoperative care resulting in unnecessary pain for about 9½ hours, while his lung was collapsing.

The Arkansas Supreme Court affirmed the trial court decision saying that the patient failed to prove that the physicians or hospital were negligent. Expert witnesses testified that it was impossible to tell how deep the brachial plexus and lung were below the surface because the thickness of the overlying soft tissue varied. The court found that none of the parties were negligent.

Napier v. Northern, 572 S.W. 2d 153 Arkansas Sup Ct (1978)

Several states have statutes defining the law of informed consent. New York Public Health Law is an example of these.

New York Public Health Law. Art. 28, Hospitals 2805 d, Limitations of Medical Malpractice Action Based on lack of Informed Consent, Amended L. 1975

1. Lack of informed consent means the failure of the person providing the professional treatment or diagnosis to disclose to the patient such alternatives thereto and the reasonably foreseeable risks and benefits involved as a reasonable medical practitioner would have disclosed in a manner permitting the patient to make a knowledgeable evaluation.
2. The right of action to recover medical malpractice based on a lack of informed consent is limited to those cases involving either (a) nonemergency treatment, procedure, or surgery, or (b) a diagnostic procedure which involves invasion of the integrity of the body.
3. For a cause of action thereto it must also be established that a reasonably prudent person in the patient's position would not have undergone the treatment or diagnosis if he had been fully informed and that the lack of informed consent is a proximate cause of the injury or condition for which recovery is sought.

4. It shall be a defense to any action for medical malpractice based on alleged failure to obtain an informed consent that:
   a. The risk not disclosed is too commonly known to warrant disclosure; or
   b. The patient assured the medical practictioner he would undergo the treatment, procedure, or diagnosis regardless of the risk involved, or the patient assured the medical practitioner he did not want to be informed of the matters to which he would be entitled to be informed; or
   c. Consent by or on behalf of the patient was not reasonably possible; or
   d. The medical practitioner, after considering all of the facts and circumstances, used reasonable discretion as to the manner and extent to which such alternatives or risks were disclosed to the patient because he reasonably believed that the manner and extent of such disclosure could reasonably be expected to adversely and substantially affect the patient's condition.

REFERENCES

1. Schoendorf V: Society of New York Hospital. 211 N.Y. 125 105 N.E. 92, 1914
2. Quimby C: Law for the Medical Practitioner. Washington AUPHA Press, 1979, p 3
3. California Hospital Association: Consent Manual. 1979, p 3
4. California Civil Code: Section 34.6, 8 & 35
5. Cobbs v. Grant 502 P. 2 d 104, Cal Rptr 505 1972

5
Negligence

If a patient suffers harm from the actions of a nurse anesthetist or any other health care professional, the legal theory that usually applies is the tort concept of negligence. Tort law recognizes the responsibility of an individual to act as an "ordinary, reasonable person" would under similar circumstances. A deviation from or breach of this reasonable person standard is considered actionable under the legal rules of negligence. The term "malpractice" has been used to encompass all liability-producing conduct by professionals. The terminology "professional negligence," has also been suggested because it has less of a negative impact.

Although the medical profession has been particularly critical of the legal profession for pursing litigation in personal injury cases resulting from medical care, there is no question that professional negligence or malpractice does occur. It has been suggested by King that there are three interested parties in a malpractice case, the patient, the health care provider, and the public.[1] The aggrieved patient seeks redress for what he or she believes to be a needless injury that may have resulted in permanent disability. The health care provider becomes defensive because of the challenge to his professional competence and the possible financial impact of an adverse judgment. Consumers have a definite interest in the medical malpractice field because the ultimate costs filter down to them through taxes and higher medical charges.

Nurse anesthetists are in no way immune from being held responsible for their professional actions, and for that reason they should have a thorough understanding of the principles of tort law that apply to their practice. No clear-cut distinctions on the standard of care for nurse anesthetists compared to physcian anesthesiologists have been identified by the courts. In other words, the standard will be the same, regardless of who administers the anesthetic. For that reason, no differentiation will be made when applying the concepts of negligence in this book between nurse anesthetists and medical anesthesia.

In an action for negligence the following components must be present and established by the plaintiff: breach, duty, standard of care, causation, and damages. Each of these elements will be considered separately and will be correlated to nurse anesthesia practice whenever possible.

DUTY

In order to be held liable for professional negligence, it must first be established that the nurse anesthetist or other health care provider owed a *duty* to the injured party. Much has been written in medical malpractice literature about whether the duty to undertake care of the patient is based on a physician-patient contract, or a traditional professional relationship.

Under the contract theory, when a physician, hospital, nurse anesthetist, or other health care professional agrees to care for a patient in exchange for a specific fee, a contractual agreement may be created with its accompanying rights and liabilities. A professional relationship is established, the "undertaking" theory holds, when a physician assumes the care of the patient.

Most of the case law regarding initiation of legal duty has pertained to either physicians or hospitals. Nurse anesthetists, particularly those employed in free-lance situations, could be found to have a legal duty under either of the prevailing theories. Hospital-employed nurse anesthetists generally do not enter into a contractual relationship with patients that is separate from the arrangements of the hospital.

Does a nurse anesthetist have a duty *not* to provide care for a patient under certain circumstances? Unfortunately, there are no cases that adequately answer this from a legal perspective. Common

Negligence

sense and accepted anesthesia practice dictate that certain patients, particularly those scheduled for elective surgery, should not receive an anesthetic until properly prepared for the procedure. If no legal duty has been established between the patient and the nurse anesthetist, it would be difficult to establish liability if damage occurred.

The following hypothetical situation is an example of the "no duty" rule that could be applied to nurse anesthetists.

Mrs. R. was admitted to the hospital for a face lift. She had no lab work, history, physical examination, or ECG. She also had eaten a large breakfast before coming to the hospital. Because she was very nervous, she demanded that a general anesthesetic be administered.

The nurse anesthetist refused to get involved in the care of the patient because the patient had not been properly prepared. The surgeon administered heavy sedation to the patient and she was monitored by the circulating nurse. Under the sedation, the patient's airway became obtunded, followed by vomiting and aspiration.

Since the nurse anesthetist refused to care for the patient, no duty was established, thus no liability could be found. The surgeon and possibly the circulating nurse could be found liable in a negligence action.

When the professional-patient relationship is prematurely terminated and causes harm to the patient, there may be liability to abandonment. The plaintiff generally must prove that the abandonment was the cause of the alleged injury.

An important court case addressed termination of professional relationship during anesthesia.

The facts as reported in the court decision indicated that the patient was an 18-year-old female admitted to Columbia Hospital for Women in Washington, D.C. for dilatation and curettage. Pentothal® (thiopental) was administered and shortly thereafter the patient developed a laryngospasm. Attempts to relax the spasm manually and by injections were unsuccessful. An endotracheal tube was inserted, but the patient was cyanotic, hypotensive, and ultimately had severe disabling brain damage.

There was considerable dispute regarding the presence of the anesthesiologist in the operating room at the time of the incident. The anesthesiologist claimed he left the OR shortly after injecting Pentothal®, but only after being relieved by another anesthesiologist. The plaintiff showed that the other anesthesiologist was administering an anesthetic in another section of the hospital when the incident occurred and could not have relieved on the case.

The court ruled that once a physician enters into a professional relationship with a patient, he is not at liberty to terminate the relationship at will. The relationship will continue until it is ended by one of the following circumstances: (1) the patient's lack of need for further care, or (2) the withdrawal of the physician upon being replaced by an equally qualified physician. The court ruled that withdrawal from the case under other circumstances constitutes a wrongful abandonment of the patient and if the patient suffers any injury as a proximate result of such abandonment, the physician is liable.

The plaintiff was awarded $1,550,000.

Ascher v. Gutierrez U.S. Ct. of Appeals, 175 U.S. App. D.C. 100 533 F 2d 1235 (1976)

The duty of the physician to verify the identity of a patient, and not assign that responsibility to other personnel, was reinforced in the following California case.

An abortion was mistakenly performed after the clerical staff confused the identity of two patients. The court noted that a physician has a professional duty to identify a surgical patient before operating and ruled that the use of nonphysician clerical help cannot alter the nondelegatable duty.

Northern Insurance Co. of New York v. Superior Court, 91 Cal. App 3d 154 Cal. Rptr 198 (1979)

Although lines of responsibility for care of equipment in hospitals are not always clear, every anesthetist has a duty to ascertain that anesthesia equipment is properly maintained before use. In the following New York case, the court ruled that the duty for maintenance of the anesthesia machine did not extend to the OR supervisor or chief of engineering.

Nitrous oxide and oxygen lines were improperly crossed, causing the patient to die of anoxia and nitrous oxide poisoning.

The legal action was against the director of nursing practice of the operating rooms, an anesthesia technician, the chief of engineering, and maintenance of the hospital. It was alleged that the anesthesia technician and the OR supervisor failed to make proper preoperative checks and inspection of the machine and failed to recognize and act upon the signs of anoxia and nitrous oxide poisoning. The chief of engineering was named for failure to properly inspect and maintain the machine, failure to follow directions and to pay attention to instructions in maintaining and repairing the machine, and crossing or permitting the nitrous oxide and oxygen lines to be crossed or mistakenly used.

The complaint was dismissed by the court which held that "none of the defendants had duties which carried with them the responsibility for the operation, use, or maintenance of the anesthesia machines in the operating room."

Hawkins v. McCluskey, 434 NYS 2d 493 New York (1981)

STANDARD OF CARE

Negligence law in general presupposes some uniform standards of behavior against which a defendant's conduct is to be evaluated.[2] Members of the health care professions are expected to possess skill and knowledge in the practice of their profession beyond that of ordinary individuals and to act in a manner consistent with that added capability.

Formulation of the standard of care by which a nurse anesthetist is evaluated is complex. One of the identifying characteristics of any professional group is its inherent right to direct and control its activities. While the professional organization of nurse anesthetists may have established and published standards of practice, legal reality may force the anesthetists to adhere to standards established by physicians. The standards by which a nurse anesthetist will be judged usually come from expert testimony and standards established by the profession.

Expert Testimony

The judicial system recognizes that juries are composed of lay people with limited or no knowledge of medical activities. For that reason, expert witnesses who are members of the profession are asked to testify as to the standard of care. The rationale being that all professionals should be held to the same level of skill which is normally prevalent among their peers.[3] The use of expert witnesses will be discussed in more detail later in the chapter.

Professional Standards

The AANA has formulated and published standards of practice for the profession. It is likely that their standards would be admitted into evidence in a negligence action and, while not conclusive of the standards of practice, would carry some authority. Copies of the standards may be obtained from the American Association of Nurse Anesthetists, 216 Higgins Road, Park Ridge, Illinois 60600.

Locality Rule

Historically, the defined standards of care for the medical profession was limited to a geographic setting. This narrow ruling indicated that one had to practice in terms of the practice in the community. The strict locality rules proved to be impractical and severely limited the pool of expert witnesses. The courts considered the fact that modern communications have expanded access to information and modified the rule to include practice in the "same or a similar locality."

In more recent years, the locality rules have undergone continued scrutiny by the courts and in a number of jurisdictions the standard has been expanded to a national level rather than local. Several anesthesia cases have been quoted in the development of national standards. In Los Alamos Medical Center, Inc. v. Coe (58 N.M. 686, 275 P. 2d 175, 1954), the court ruled that the standard of care for administering morphine is the same regardless of locality. In Webb v. Jones (488 S.W. 2d 407, Texas, 1972), the court said: ". . . given human tolerance levels for anesthetics, there are certain minimum procedures required regardless of locality to insure proper levels of vaporization of the anesthetic."

The following, Burne v. Belinkoff, is the leading anesthetic case that abolished the locality rule.

The plaintiff asked for recovery of damages from the defendant because of alleged negligence in administering a spinal anesthetic.

The defendant anesthesiologist administered a spinal anesthetic to the patient for a delivery. The drugs used were Pontocaine® [tetracaine] 8 mg in 1 cc glucose 10 percent. When the plaintiff attempted to get out of bed 11 hours later, she slipped and fell to the floor. The plaintiff subsequently complained of numbness and weakness in her left leg which persisted at the time of the trial.

Trial testimony given by eight physicians related to the patient's condition and evidence that her condition resulted from an excessive dosage of Pontocaine®. There was evidence that the dosage was customary in New Bedford, Massachusetts, the location of the incident.

The court overruled the locality rule and a more global standard of practice be applied.

Burne v. Belinkoff, 354 MA 102, 235 N.E. 2d 793 (1968)

CAUSATION

In malpractice actions the plaintiff must establish that the alleged negligent act of the defendant caused the injury. This element of negligence, called "causation," is an important factor in malpractice cases. Proof of causation may be based upon direct testimony, usually by the use of expert witnesses.

The two most common tests to establish causation are classified as "but for" and "substantial factor." In the former, the plaintiff must prove that it was more probably true than not that the patient's injury would not have occurred "but for" the defendant's action. The latter test requires that the defendant's conduct was a "substantial factor" in producing the injury.[4]

The standard most commonly applied to causation requires that the patient's injury has been "more likely than not" the result of the defendant's conduct.

Multiple causation can present difficulties in malpractice cases. The cause of the injury frequently is not easily determined to be due to one single factor. An example of this can be seen in anesthesia cases where a patient dies from hypovolemia. Was the cause of the death due to errors in surgical technique or failure of the anesthetist to adequately monitor and replace lost fluid? A plaintiff's attorney usually will attempt to ascertain multiple causation, so that many defendants will be contributing to the damage awards.

The following case illustrates application of the concept of causation in anesthesia suits.

In June, 1975, the patient underwent surgery to excise lymph nodes in his right groin and right armpit. As a result of that surgery, he alleged that he suffered damage to the median ulnar nerves due to the surgeon's negligence. He also sued the anesthestist, recovery room nurse, and hospital, alleging that his left eye had been injured when a foreign substance was dropped into it by the anesthetist immediately before or during surgery.

The court trial resulted in a directed verdict in favor of all the defendants and the case was dismissed. The appellate court upheld the defense verdict and said that the ". . . plaintiff produced no proof of any causual connection between his alleged eye injury and (the) defendants' actions. . . . (We) conclude that the evidence offered was woefully insufficient to connect the plaintiff's eye injury to the defendants."

Regas v. Argonaut Southern Insurance Co. et al., CA. App. 379 So 2d 822 (1980)

In another case, the application of the concept of negligence is illustrated.

A 32-year-old, healthy patient underwent gall bladder surgery. During the process of removing the gall bladder, the surgeon noted an abnormally short cystic duct that was embedded in the liver. The surgeon removed a small wedge of the common bile duct and then attempted to repair it. A stab wound was made and the inferior portion of the raw liver began bleeding. The surgeon attempted to control the bleeding by applying posterior pressure to the vena cava.

The anesthesiologist, noticing the bleeding, ordered extra units of blood and requested that an ECG monitor be brought in. Even though the patient received blood, her blood pressure dropped and she eventually suffered a cardiac arrest. An assistant surgeon began cardiac massage and was able to restore function, but the patient never awoke from a coma.

In the medical malpractice action, the appellate court upheld the jury verdict for the plaintiff. They found that the evidence was factually and legally sufficient to support the jury's finding that the anesthesiologist's *negligence in failing to timely recognize the patient's cardiac arrest was a proximate cause of her death.*

Garza v. Berlanga, Texas Civil Appeal 598 S.W. 2d 377, (1980)

The following case illustrates multiple defendants and the issue of causation.

The patient was admitted to the hospital May, 1968 for elective surgery on her submaxillary gland. Endotracheal intubation was difficult and was successful only after two attempts by an anesthesiologist, after two other attempts by the anesthesia resident had failed. The time from induction to intubation was about 20 minutes. About 5 minutes after intubation, the surgeon noted that the patient was cyanotic. The chief anesthesiologist entered the room and while he was working on the patient, the surgeon left the OR. After 5 minutes, while the anesthesiologist was preparing to check the endotracheal tube, the patient suffered a cardiac arrest. He immediately removed the tube and the surgeon began external heart massage. The patient's skin color and heartbeat returned to normal, but she had already suffered permanent brain damage.

Negligence

The ensuing legal action brought about a jury verdict of $1,000,000 for the patient's husband and $500,000 for the patient. The appellate court upheld the trial court decision and on the issue of causation said that the *surgeon's conduct had been a proximate cause of the patient's injuries.*

At the trial, the expert witness testified that the surgeon should have given orders to cancel the anesthesia when it was apparent the patient was in trouble. The hospital and chief anesthesiologist were also found negligent.

Schneider v. Albert Einstein Medical Center, North Division, 390 A. 2d 1271 Pa. (1978)

DAMAGES

The final element necessary for actionable negligence is *damages*. This term generally refers to the loss or injury suffered. Damages are usually categorized as nominal, compensatory, and punitive.

Nominal damages refer to a very small amount of money awarded to a party where there is no substantial loss or injury to be compensated, but rather only a technical invasion of the plaintiff's protected rights.

Compensatory damages, the type most frequently awarded in medical professional negligence cases, consist of the acutal loss suffered. The purpose of compensatory damages is to make an appropriate, and usually counterbalancing payment to the plaintiff for an actual loss or injury sustained through the act or default of the defendant, thereby "making the plaintiff whole" as much as possible. General and special damages are components of compensatory damages. General damages are those that flow from the wrong complained of and are often known as "pain and suffering." Special damages are the actual monetary value of the negligent act and are reflected in such awards as additional money for hospital bills because of anticipated custodial care for the life of the injured party.

Punitive or exemplary damages are awarded as punishment to the defendants for acts the jury considers to be aggravated, willful, or wanton. Punitive damages are awarded or withheld at the discretion of the jury.

Wrongful Death

When a patient dies as the result of negligent acts of a health care provider, the survivors may collect for wrongful death. A number of states have wrongful death statutes that establish the basis for recovery and the maximum amount of damages that may be recovered.

The issue of recovery for loss of life's pleasures and amenities in a wrongful death action were adddresed in this Pennsylvania case involving a nurse anesthetist.

A 5-year-old child, in excellent health, was admitted to the hospital for a T & A. A nurse anesthetist supervised by an anesthesiologist administered the anesthetic. During the procedure, the anesthesiologist was called to an emergency in another OR. When he returned, he noticed that the child was cyanotic with no apparent heartbeat. The nurse anesthetist was still administering a full concentration of anesthetic agent and was not using precordial monitoring. Emergency resuscitation restored the patient's heartbeat, but, because of the prolonged cardiac arrest, he suffered severe brain damage and died about 7 weeks later.

The child's father filed suit on behalf of his son's estate for wrongful death. The jury awarded the estate $455,199 and the hospital appealed.

The Pennsylvania Supreme Court said that "the trial judge erred in instructing the jury on the amount of damages. The trial court had instructed the jury that it could consider pain and suffering and compensation for loss of future earnings and loss of amenities or pleasures of life. In the higher court's ruling, they said *loss of life's pleasures or amenities was not one of the elements of recovery for wrongful death and survival action* [author's emphasis]."

Willinger v. Mercy Catholic Medical Center of Southern Pennsylvania, 393 A 2d 1188 Pa. (1978)

The amount of damages to be awarded against a surgeon who operated on the wrong patient was at issue in the following Kentucky case.

The patient, Gladys Bruce, was scheduled for a conization of the cervix. She had an identification bracelet on her wrist, but none of the parties involved checked her identification with her bracelet. Since Mrs. Bruce answered to the name of "Smith," a patient scheduled for a thyroidectomy, the surgeon proceeded with a thyroidectomy on Mrs. Bruce. When it was realized that she was the wrong patient, the incision was closed.

Mrs. Bruce brought legal action against the hospital, anesthesiologist, surgical technician, and surgeon for malpractice. The court ruled that the fact that the patient answered to the name of another patient did not excuse the failure of the surgeon, anesthesiologist, and surgical technician to determine the identity of the patient by examining her identification bracelet.

The following damages were awarded: $10,000 against the surgeon and $90,000 against the hospital, anesthesiologist, and surgical technician.

Southeastern Kentucky Baptist v. Bruce Ky., 539 S.W. 286 (1976)

PROVING PROFESSIONAL NEGLIGENCE

Except for certain exceptions, expert testimony is required to establish the appropriate standard of care in professional negligence cases. Both the plaintiff and the defendant rely on the testimony of expert witnesses to prove or to defend their case. Experts may also be used to determine causation and damages.

In order to qualify as an expert witness, a person must possess qualification and be knowledgable in the area in question. The Federal Rules of Evidence indicate that an expert be qualified by "knowledge, skill, experience, training, and education."[5]

As is apparent to even the most casual observer, anesthesiologists are used as expert witnesses in cases involving nurse anesthetists. In other words, the standard of care for anesthesia in court cases, appears to be established almost exclusively by anesthesiologists rather than nurse anesthetists. Although there is a growing trend of nurse anesthetists acting as expert witnesses, the use of anesthesiologists for this purpose is still the most common practice. Nurse anesthetists, in the spirit of professionalism, have an obligation to be willing to verify standards of care by offering expert testimony.

POSSIBLE EXCEPTIONS TO EXPERT WITNESS REQUIREMENT

As previously mentioned, expert testimony is the primary method of establishing the standard of care for professionals. There are, however, exceptions to this rule that have a direct application to nurse anesthesia practice. One of these is "common knowledge." This rule recognizes that under certain circumstances lay people can recognize negligence without the guidance of experts. A case in which the common knowledge concept was employed involved burns on the patient's buttocks following vascular surgery (Wiles v. Myerly, 210 N.W. 2d 619 Iowa 1973). Another case centered on the question of whether a postoperative pateint's acute condition required notificaiton of the patient's attending physician (Karrigan v. Nazareth Convent & Academy, Inc., 212 Kan 44, 510 P. 2d 190, 1973).

The following case concerning dental anesthesia illustrates how the common knowledge exception to expert testimony was applied.

The patient was an obese, middle-aged woman who suffered from hypertension, a systolic heart murmur, and chronic myocarditis. She visited a dentist to have a filling replaced.

The dentist injected Xylocaine® [lidocaine] with epinephrine into her gums. She asked him to wait a few minutes as she was "very nervous." He waited 3–4 minutes, began work, and completed filling the tooth in about 20 minutes. The patient rose from the dental chair and fell, having suffered a cerebral hemmorhage. She died 3 days later.

In the negligence action the patient's family claimed the defendant deviated from the standard of care among dentists by failing to take a medical history before administering anesthesia. The defendant-dentist said that it was his "guess" that he had asked the patient about her general health, but his chart contained no notation about her health problems.

The higher court held that a jury could reasonably conclude that the defendant knew or should have known that it was dangerous to administer epinephrine to a hypertensive patient. The court held that it was within *common knowlege of laymen* that a reasonable man, including the dentist, who knows a drug is potentially harmful to a certain type of patient should take adequate precaution before administering the drug or deciding whether to administer it.

Sanzari v. Rosenfeld, Supt Ct N.J. 34 128, 167 A 2d 624 (1961)

PACKAGE INSERTS AND MANUFACTURERS' INSTRUCTIONS

Whether package inserts of drugs or manufacturers' instructions regarding use of equipment should be admissible as evidence of the standard of care is an interesting and complex question. It is often common practice to use drugs in ways that deviate from the package inserts. The clinician is well aware that package inserts and other drug information protect the manufacturer and can be interpreted as being restrictive in practical situations.

Most courts hold that manufacturers' recommendations are at least admissible as evidence of the standard of care. However, they have seldom, if ever, been considered conclusive. A number of courts have upheld the admissibility of manufacturers' instructions where they are properly validated or refuted by an expert witness.

A liberal approach to this subject was adopted in a Minnesota case where the court held:

"When drug manufacturers recommend to the medical profession (1) the conditions under which the drug should be prescribed; (2) the disorder it is designed to relieve; (3) the precautionary measures which should be observed; and (4) warns of the dangers that are inherent in its use, a doctor's deviation from such recommendations is *prima facie* evidence of negligence if there is competent medical testimony that his patient's injury or death resulted from the doctor's failure to adhere to the recommendations. Under such circumstances it is incumbent on the doctor to disclose his reasons for departing from the procedures recommended by the manufacturer."

Mulder v. Parke Davis & Co., 288 Minn. 332, 340, 181 N.W. 2d 882, 887 (1970).

It appears that most courts would not accept a manufacturer's recommendations and package inserts as conclusive evidence of the standard of care. Although the instructions would probably be admitted into evidence, expert witnesses would be called for reinforcement as to the standard of practice.

MEDICAL LITERATURE

The rules of evidence clearly regard the use of textbooks, periodicals, and other literature as hearsay; thus medical literature is not admissible as direct evidence to prove the statements it contains. The arguments against using this literature for establishing conclusive evidence of the standard of care are many and include the following: (1) the author may not be present; (2) there is no opportunity for cross examination; and (3) the literature may be out of date.

It has been recommended that a more sensible view would be to hold medical literature as admissible under limited circumstances.

Where a conflict exists between the medical treatise and the professional standards established by expert witnesses, a good approach would be to hold both sources admissible as evidence. The jury or the judge would then determine which source was most probative.[1]

A Louisiana case illustrates how one court viewed use of package inserts as evidence of the standard of care.

A nurse anesthetist was sued by a patient for physical complications, including phlebitits and thrombosis of the arm from improper administration of Valium® [diazepam]. At the trial it was established that the manufacturer's recommendation for Valium® administration is that the drug should be ". . . administered slowly, taking 1 minute for each 5 mg given. . . ."

Medical experts stated that the anesthetist adhered to proper standards of medical practice. The anesthetist testified that she always administered Valium® slowly in order to judge its effect. She also testified that she did not administer the Valium® to the patient any faster than she administered it at any other time and that she always administered it in general conformity with the manufacturer's recommendations. She did not use a watch to time the injection.

Expert testimony verified that to use a watch was not the standard of practice and that specialists do not follow manufacturers' inserts concerning the administration of Valium® or other medications strictly or literally. Therefore, even if the anesthetist did not administer the Valium® in the precise time directed in the manufacturer's insert, her degree of precision and care did not vary from that adhered to in her field of specialty and that she did not breach the malpractice statute.

The appellate court supported the finding that the nurse anesthetist acted in accordance with accepted medical practice in administering injectable Valium.®

Mohr v. Jenkins, 393 So 2d 245 LA, (1980)

RES IPSA LOQUITUR

Professional negligence can be proved by either direct evidence which delineates the act and explains why it was negligent or, in certain circumstances, by indirect evidence (circumstantial) under the doctrine of *res ipsa loquitur*.

Res ipsa loquitur translates literally as "the thing speaks for itself." Negligence may be inferred from the fact of an unexplained

Negligence

injury that does not normally occur in the absence of negligence. *Res ipsa loquitur* is often pleaded in anesthesia cases, particularly when a healthy patient is injured during an anesthetic procedure. The rationale of the plaintiff's attorney is that there must have been negligence otherwise the patient would not have been injured. Examples of both successful and unsuccessful holdings on this doctrine will be presented later in this chapter.

Elements

For the doctrine of *res ipsa loquitiur* to apply, three elements generally must be present. They can be summarized as follows: (1) The event must be of a kind which ordinarily does not occur in the absence of negligence. (2) It must be caused by an agency or instrumentality within the exclusive control of the defendant. (3) It must not have been due to any voluntary action or contributory action on the part of the plaintiff.

It is important to understand that the doctrine of *res ipsa loquitur* does not automatically apply because of an unsatisfactory result. There must not only have been an unfortunate result, but there must also be a rational basis for inferring that such a result does not normally occur in the absence of negligence.

A large number of anesthesia cases utilizing a *res ipsa loquitur* pleading are those in which patients have received nerve damage, either from alleged improper postioning or from regional anesthesia. Although cases of cardiac arrest may also apply under a *res ipsa* holding, a number of courts have denied use of the doctrine in these cases.

A child brought suit against the hospital, surgeon, and anesthesiologist to recover damages for facial scars allegedly sustained during an operation to excise the child's tonsils and adnoids. The 5-year-old awoke from the surgery with blisters on her face. The blebs ruptured and, upon healing, noticeable scars remained. The scars, the suit claimed, were a source of anxiety and the cause of emotional suffering to the child.

The plaintiff's attorneys at the time of the trial were cognizant of the fact that the child was unconscious during the operation and thus unable to relate the events that produced the blisters which resulted in the scarring. Moreover, they did not produce expert witnesses who might have given the opinion that the scars were the direct result of negligent treatment.

The court of special appeal held that the child had failed to prove that any of the defendants had exclusive control of the instruments which caused the injury, thus the requisites for invocation of *res ipsa loquitur* were not fulfilled.

Stevens v. Union Memorial Hospital, Md. App 424 A 2d 118 (1981)

The following case is another illustration of the court's denial of the *res ipsa* doctrine.

An 11-year-old male in otherwise good health was scheduled for elective surgery to correct a pectus excavation, July, 1975. At the commencement of the operation, a heart block occurred. All the usual drug and closed heart massage techniques failed to restore the heartbeat. The patient suffered severe brain damage from anoxia and died 3 days later.

The parents filed a wrongful death claim against the hospital, six physicians, and a nurse anesthetist—all of whom were involved in the operation. The trial court dismissed the case against the parties and the parents appealed.

The appellate court said that the parents had not proved that cardiac arrest was not the kind of injury that normally occurred in the absence of negligence. They ruled that *res ipsa loquitur* did not apply to the case for the additional reason that there was an absence of direct evidence to explain the activities leading to the cardiac arrest.

Ewen v. Baton Rouge General Hospital, So 2d LA Ct of App (1979)

The following is a case where the *res ipsa* doctrine was not upheld but the plaintiff collected damages.

A nurse anesthetist positioned a patient's left arm containing the I.V. infusion on an armboard. Upon awakening in the recovery room following surgery, the patient experienced severe pain in her neck, left shoulder, and left arm. This pain was diagnosed as resulting from a suprascapular nerve palsy allegedly caused by the malpositioning of the patient.

The trial court awarded a verdict of $56,000, and found the physician, nurse anesthetist, and hospital liable. The appeal court did not uphold the *res ipsa loquitur* holding against the physician for the reason that the patient failed to eliminate other responsible causes.

Jones v. Harrisburg Polyclinic Hosptial, 410 A. 2d 303 PA Super (1979)

Other cases involving *res ipsa loquitur* holdings will be found in the following chapter in the section on regional anesthesia.

Negligence

DEFENSES TO NEGLIGENCE

In any civil action seeking damages for personal injuries or wrongful death, there is no presumption of innocence. The trial of a medical malpractice action requires the defendant to attempt to meet and refute the plaintiff's allegations on the merits of the case. There are certain substantative defenses that apply to medical malpractice actions, including the statute of limitations, contributory negligence, Good Samaritan defense, indemnity, arbitration agreement, and Workmen's Compensation laws.

Statute of Limitations

As a result of the "medical malpractice crisis" in the mid 1970s, a number of state legislatures enacted changes in laws applying to malpractice limitations. The general rule of a statute of limitations is that unless an action is commenced within a prescribed period of time, it will not be heard.

Most laws covering statutes of limitations in medical cases rely on what is known as the *discovery rule*. This rule usually provides that an action for medical malpractice originates when the plaintiff discovers or should have discovered the injury. Many of the discovery rule cases were inspired by medical injuries that were difficult to discover, such as foreign objects left in a body cavity during surgery. An example is found in Flanagan v. General Hospital (24 NY 2d 427, 301 NYS 2d 23, 1969). The plaintiff had an operation on July 14, 1958 during which time surgical clamps were inadvertently left in his body. The patient was advised of this circumstance in June, 1966 when x-rays revealed the clamps. He required another operation for their removal. The court ruled that in situations where a foreign object is left in a patient's body, it cannot be claimed that the patient's action is feigned or frivolous. In addition, there is no possible causal break between the negligence of the doctor or hospital and the patient's injury. The statute of limitations in the Flanagan case did not apply,

The so-called discovery rule employed in foreign object medical malpractice cases is in harmony with the purpose for which statutes of limitations were enacted and strikes a fair balance in the field of medical malpractice. The court noted that the clamps, though immersed within the patient's body and undiscovered for a long period of time, retained their identity so that the defendant's ability to defend a "stale" claim was not unduly impaired. As such, when a foreign object has negligently been left in the patient's body, the statute of limitations will not begin to run until the patient could have reasonably discovered the malpractice. A synopsis of statutes of limitation for each state is found in the appendix.

Contributory-Comparative Negligence

If any act or omission on the part of the patient contributed to or caused his own injury, aggravated or exacerbated the injury or disability, then an affirmative defense of contributing or comparative negligence is pleaded. The difference between contributing and comparative negligence is that, in states where the former is followed, a finding of contributory negligence will completely bar the plaintiff's recovery. In comparative negligence jurisdictions, a percentage of the plaintiff's injury will be used to reduce or mitigate the award.

An anesthesia case that illustrates the defense of contributory negligence follows:

The patient had been taking Lasix® [furosemide], a strong diuretic prior before her admission to the hospital for a breast biopsy. She had a cardiac arrest under anesthesia. Normal heart function was restored with difficulty and brain damage resulted.

The doctors contended that the patient gave a false history regarding use of the drug and, as a result, they proceeded without taking any precautions to avoid the risks incident to a low potassium level. While both defendant physicians denied receiving any history of the patient's use of Lasix®, such information was given by the patient to a nurse who did not record it in her notes. The plaintiff contended that the defendants knew, or by the exercise of ordinary care should have known, that she was using Lasix®.

In affirming the jury verdict in favor of the physicians, the appeals court said: "For his own safety, a patient must exercise ordinary care to give an accurate history to his treating physician. He must tell the truth. Otherwise, the patient may mislead the physician, with disastrous results. Because the patient's self interest dictates that he tell the truth, the history given the physician is deemed particularly reliable, and it is admissible into evidence as an exception to the hearsay rule, In determining what constitutes contributory negligence in giving a history, consideration must be given to the special relationship that exists between patient and physician."

The court also said that although there was no direct evidence that the patient knew she was suffering from a pre-existing heart condition, the circumstantial evidence supported a conclusion that she did know. Her actions mislead the physicians and were a substantial factor in her cardiac arrest.

Mackey v. Greenview Hosp. Inc., 587 S.W. 2d 249 Ky. Ct of App. (1979)

Good Samaritan Statute

There is a good samaritan statute in all 50 states and the District of Columbia. Originally enacted by the California legislature in 1959, the statutes are intended to protect the physician or medical care provider who acts as a good samaritan from tort liability.

Most states have included a *good faith* requirement in their good samaritan laws. Under this rule a person will not be held liable for ordinary negligence providing he acted in good faith when giving aid, and was not guilty of gross, willful, or wanton negligence. A recent California case expands good samaritan immunity to the hospital.

A hospital resident responded to an emergency and administered certain therapy in an attempt to reverse a cardiac arrest. The hospital resident and the hospital were sued under the doctrine of *respondeat superior,* The hospital contended that the physician was a volunteer and had no legal duty to respond to the emergency signal; he was not on call for emergencies and as such was not a member of the hospital team whose duties included responding to such emergencies.

In affirming a verdict for the defendants, the appellate court noted that the need to encourage physicians to render emergency care, when they otherwise might not, must prevail over the policy of vindicating the rights of the malpractice victim.

McKenna v. Cedars of Lebanon Hospital, 93 Cal. App 3d 282, 155 Cal. Rptr 631 (1979)

REFERENCES

1. King J: The Law of Medical Malpractice. St. Paul, West Publishing Co, 1974
2. Prosser W: Law of Torts, 149, ed 4. 1971
3. Kucera W: Sources of the standards of care in malpractice actions. AANA J, April, p 184–186, 1976
4. Restatement, Second Torts, 431 Cal. 432, 1965
5. Federal Rules of Evidence, 702

6
Anesthesia Practice and Lawsuits

The major concern of any clinician, whether physician or nurse anesthetist, is the safety of the patient. Medical personnel resent legal influence on clinical practice, but the facts and statistics clearly indicate that serious mishaps occur under anesthesia, causing death or serious bodily harm to the patient. If these mishaps are caused by negligence, the remedy available to the patient is often found in the legal system.

All anesthetists have a duty to their patients, to themselves, and their profession to carefully evaluate their clinical practice from the perspective of preventing anesthesia accidents that could harm a patient and potentially lead to a lawsuit. This chapter identifies critical incidents and preventable anesthesia mishaps, and illustrates them with case examples, to assist the anesthetist in evaluating his or her practice.

Unfortunately, even in the best practice situations, anesthesia and surgical accidents do occur. Anesthetists may be placed in the situation of having to defend their actions. An ounce of preventative medicine, by means of accurate record keeping and maintaining the state of the art, will be very beneficial in defending a lawsuit should an accident occur.

The first recorded death from anesthesia occurred in New Castle, England on January 28, 1847. The patient was a healthy 15-year-old girl who was to have a toenail removed. A surgeon administered the chloroform anesthetic and described the incident as follows:

"She appeared to dread the operation and fretted a great deal. . . . The inhalation . . . was done from a handkerchief on which a teaspoonful of chloroform had been poured. After drawing her breath twice, she pulled my hand from her mouth. I told her to put her hands on her knees and to breath quietly, which she did. In about half a minute, seeing no change in breathing or alteration of pulse, I lifted her arm, which I found rigid. I looked at the pupil and pinched her cheek and, finding her insensible, requested Mr. Lloyd to begin the operation. At the termination of the semilunar incision she gave a kick or twitch, which caused me to think the chloroform had not sufficient effect. I was proceeding to apply more to the handkerchief when her lips, which had previously been of a good color, became suddenly blanched, and she spluttered at her mouth as if in epilepsy. I threw down the handkerchief and dashed cold water in her face, and gave her some internally, followed by brandy, without, however, the least effect, not the slightest attempt at a rally being made. We laid her on the floor, opened a vein in her arm, and the jugular vein, but no blood flowed. The whole process of inhalation, operation, venesection, and death, could not, I should say, have occupied more than 2 minutes."[1]

Statistics of malpractice claims from anesthesia accidents are not readily available for several reasons: insurance companies are somewhat reluctant to release information regarding claims, anesthetists do not freely offer facts about suits, and a large number of suits get settled out of court. Legal literature, therefore, does not accurately reflect statistics.

INA Loss Control Services Inc., the insurance company sponsored by the AANA, has reported claims for the period of September, 1978 to September, 1979 (Table 6-1).[2] Identification of the

Table 6-1
Claims and Incidents Reported by the INA from September, 1978 to September, 1979 by Type of Injury*

Type of Injury	Number	Percent
Death	20	35.1
Brain damage	3	5.3
Damage to teeth/dentures	11	19.3
Phlebitis	4	7.0
All other	19	33.0
Total	57	100

*From Althouse, J: Rx Loss Control—An Analysis of Anesthesia Related Claims. AANA J Feb, 1980, 59–60. Reprinted with permission.

Anesthesia Practice and Lawsuits

Table 6-2
Incidents and/or Claims Reported by the INA that resulted in death or brain damage with documented preanesthesia evaluation*

	Number	Percentage
With preanesthesia evaluation	8	40.0
Without preanesthesia evaluation	12	60.0
Total	20	100

*From Althouse, J: Rx Loss Control—An Analysis of Anesthesia Related Claims. AANA J Je, 1980, 277–279. Reprinted with permission.

causal factors leading to alleged malpractice is important to the anesthetist when reviewing his own practice. In cases where the injury was an anesthesia-related brain damage or death, failure to maintain intubation, failure to monitor during anesthesia, and failure in the administration of medication were identified as alleged causal factors.[3] The importance of preanesthesia evaluation was stressed by INA in a report which indicated that 60 percent of the patients with death or brain damage did not have a documented preanesthesia evaluation (Table 6-2). Cardiac arrest, adverse reaction, and teeth damage were the most three frequent allegations in anesthesia-related claims reported by the St. Paul Fire & Marine Insurance Company for the period of October, 1973 through March, 1980 (Table 6-3).[4]

How safe is anesthesia? What are the patient risks when receiving an anesthetic? Is one type of anesthetic safer than another? What are the factors that could lead to complications and ultimately

Table 6-3
Anesthesia-Related Claims Reported by the St. Paul Fire and Marine Insurance Co. from October, 1973 to March, 1980*

Claim	Number	Percentage
Cardiac Arrest	404	32
Adverse Reaction	359	29
Teeth Damage	317	25
Other Catastrophic	118	9
Other Unknown	54	4
Total	1252	99

*From Minneapolis St. Paul Fire and Marine Insurance Co: Summary of anesthesia-related malpractice claims: Malpractice Digest May/June, 1980. Reprinted with permission.

a malpractice action? A number of studies have been conducted where anesthesia mortality, morbidity, and risk factors were reported. The general conclusions indicate anesthesia to be relatively safe, but not without risk.[5-7] Factors associated with anestheia risk have been identified as human factors, operative procedures, patient disease, and age. Since anesthetics alter the normal physiology and interfere with homeostatic mechanisms, risk factors are an inherent part of any anesthetic technique.

Probable cause of unexpected cardiac arrests have been studied by several sources. Taylor and Larsen divide the causes into four categories: anesthetic mismanagement, cardiovascular abnormalties, hypoxia due to hypoventilation, and miscellaneous causes. Delay in recognizing cardiac arrest, lack of proper preanesthesia evaluation, and inadequate, immediate postoperative care were listed by Wylie in a series of 66 cases reported between 1964 and 1973.[8] Wylie concluded that cardiac arrest might have been prevented in 50 percent of the cases.

PREVENTABLE ANESTHESIA MISHAPS

Preventable anesthesia mishaps with emphasis on human factors were studied by Cooper and associates.[9] Recognizing the frequency of mishaps, when the incidents occur, and the factors most frequently associated with them can be very useful to an anesthetist in analyzing his or her own individual habits and also can be a means of decreasing the associated risks.

Certain types of errors were found to occur with relatively high frequency (Table 6-4). Cooper postulates that some errors occur with such regularity that they are now accepted as a fact of life in anesthesia. He said: "Rather than taking action to prevent recurrence, anesthetists are expected to rely purely on their own vigilance to detect the initial problem or its resultant clinical signs after the fact."[10]

The factors most frequently associated with preventable anesthesia incidents (Table 6-5) were an important aspect of Cooper's study. It would be very difficult to defend an anesthetist in a legal action if the patient's mishap was due to one of these factors. A number of legal cases reported here illustrate a variety of mishaps which lead to patient harm and ultimately a lawsuit. The following case was settled on the third day of the trial and emphasizes several of the points mentioned above.

Anesthesia Practice and Lawsuits

Table 6-4
Frequent Preventable Anesthetic Incidents*

Breathing circuit disconnection
Incorrect drug dose
Wrong gas flow setting
Syringe swap
Intravenous line disconnection
Laryngoscope malfunction
Breathing circuit misconnection
Hypovolemia
Tracheal airway device position change
Other (e.g., vial) drug swap
Ventilator malfunction

*From Cooper J: Avoiding Preventable Mishaps. Chicago, ASA Refresher Course, 1979, p 235. Reprinted with permission.

"The patient, a 36-year-old female, was hospitalized in 1935 for bilateral breast biopsy. Premedication was Seconal® [secobarbital], Demoral® [meperidine], and atropine.

"When she was brought to the OR at 7:45 A.M., an ECG monitor was attached and an I.V. line inserted. Blood pressure was recorded at 110/70 mm Hg. The following drugs were given by an anesthesiologist at 7:50 A.M.: Innovar® 2 cc and Pavulon® [pancuronium bromide] 4mg, The oxygen was

Table 6-5
Factors Most Frequently Associated with Preventable Anesthesia Incidents*

Inadequate total experience
Inadequate familiarity with equipment and/or device
Poor communication with team, lab, etc.
Haste
Inattention and/or carelessness
Fatigue
Excessive dependency on other personnel
Failure to perform proper checkout and/or history
Supervisor not present enough
Visual field restricted
Inadequate familiarity with surgical procedure
Teaching activity underway
Inadequate familiarity with anesthetic technique
"First time" incident

*From Cooper J: Avoiding Preventable Mishaps. Chicago, ASA Refresher Course, 1979, p 235. Reprinted with permission.

turned on and the mask was held at an angle to her face. At 7:55 A.M., the patient was given Pentothal® [thiopental] 5 cc and within seconds she developed a laryngospasm.

"The anesthesiologist tried unsuccessfully to insert an endotracheal tube. He told the circulating nurse to bring some Anectine® [succinylcholine chloride], but there was none in the operating room and she had to go to a cabinet outside the operating room to get it. The drug was given, the laryngospasm relieved, and the endotracheal tube inserted. While there was a transient bradycardia at the time of the intubation, there was no cardiac arrest or even a period of hypotension.

"A second problem was that the oxygen line was not connected. The anesthesiologist looked at the outlet on his machine, saw a hose draped over it and assumed the hose was connected. The nurse would sometimes make this connection for him, but it had not been made on this particular day. The error was recognized shortly after the complication occurred.

"At 8:05 A.M., another 5 cc of Pentothal® was given intravenously. The patient was observed for several minutes and because her vital signs were stable, the doctors decided to proceed with surgery. The vital sign remained stable during the procedure and the anesthesia was discontinued at the end of surgery, about 10:30 A.M. The patient was transferred to the recovery room at 10:45 A.M.

"A recovery room chart entry at 11:00 A.M. stated that the patient did not respond to painful stimuli. At 11:50 A.M., she was still not responsive, although her color had been good throughout. At 12:30 P.M., her blood pressure rose from 150/80 to 200/80 and she displayed convulsive movements. A neurosurgeon, called as a consultant, determined there was acute brain damage. An EEG revealed diffuse cerebral cortical dysfunction, consistent with hypoxia injury. The patient remained comatose for 13 days and then recovered full consciousness.

"At the time of the trial, the patient had a normal I.Q., but had slow, scanning speech and motor impairment. She spends most of her time in a wheelchair and has to be on medication to prevent siezures. The strength of the plaintiff's case was related to the delay in administering Anectine®, as well as the unconnected oxygen hose.

"The settlement was for a total of $750,000—$575,000 from the anesthesiologist's insurance carrier and $175,000 from the hospital."

Alameda Superior Court No. 466920-9, reported in Rubsamen D: Professional Liability Newsletter, January 1979. Reprinted with permission.

OBSTETRIC ANESTHESIA

Numerous legal cases involving obstetrics can be found in the legal literature. The reasons for this are obvious—bad results in obstetrics often involves both mother and baby and can produce great emotional impact. Areas of concern to the anesthetist include maternal and fetal monitoring and mortality due to anesthesia, the legality of having fathers and others in the delivery room, and consent for obstetric and related procedures.

Anesthesia continues to be implicated as a leading cause of maternal mortality. Since the pregnant parturient is known to have a full stomach, every general anesthesia technique requires the use of an endotracheal tube. It would be very difficult, perhaps impossible, to find an expert witness to testify that the standard of care in obstetrics does not include endotracheal intubation for general anesthesia. With regional anesthesia in obstetrics receiving popular acceptance with patients, their families, and hospital personnel, nurse anesthetists should be involved with that technique and aware of potential problems that might develop.

The consumer movement has brought about many changes in health care, including the presence of the father in the delivery room. While most anesthetists feel uncomfortable with the situation, there is no question that this trend is firmly established. Most hospitals have developed policies for fathers in the delivery room and request that they sign a release form. Anesthetists should familiarize themselves with the policy of their institution.

The following case presents a lawsuit that arose from the presence of the father in the delivery room when a complication developed.

> The plaintiff's wife was a patient of the defendant for the purpose of delivery of a child. The patient died during the delivery process. Plaintiff, who was inside the delivery room, was able to feel life in the unborn child. He asked the attending physician and the nurses to deliver the child, but they refused. The child died and plaintiff was able to ascertain the death by feeling his wife's body. He sued under a cause of action to recover for the emotional distress resulting from the death of his child.
>
> The court of appeals held that the plaintiff had a triable cause of action for emotional distress in that he had alleged, in addition to the other necessary elements, that he learned of the death through his own observations of the cessation of life and that his shock and distress were occasioned by that sensory and contemporaneous recognition of the death.

Austin v. The Regents of the University of California, 89 Cal. App 3d 354 (1979)

PREVENTION OF SUITS

Most hospitals have developed risk management programs, often in conjunction with their malpractice insurance carrier, where areas of high risk for lawsuits are identified and changes are implemented through a structured program. Anesthesia departments have performed the same task through chart audits, quality assurance programs, and peer reviews. Specific areas in anesthesia lawsuit prevention are in preanesthetic evaluation, use of monitoring devices, proper equiment and supplies, prevention of tooth and nerve damage, and postoperative care.

Preanesthesia Evaluation

The preanesthesia period is the logical starting point to identify potential problems that could lead to complications and resulting lawsuits. It has been well established that a thorough preanesthesia evaluation, which includes developing a good rapport with the patient, is a most effective means of establishing the nurse anesthetist as an important member of the health care team. The standards of practice for nurse anesthetists dictate that certain aspects of the preanesthesia evaluation are essential to establish an anesthesia care plan for the patient. Anesthetists who fall short in this area will find themselves in a precarious legal situation when defending a lawsuit based on failure to identify potential anesthesia risks or need for additional tests or consultation.

The patient interview presents the anesthetist with the opportunity to establish rapport with the patient. Patients should be shown understanding, sincere interest, and reassured about the care they will receive under anesthesia. Such rapport is a professional responsibility and will be a useful deterrent to future lawsuits should a bad result occur. It has been stated that patients who like their physicians rarely sue and that lack of rapport is a common denominator in many malpractice actions.[11]

After the appropriate chart review, patient interview, and physical assessment (and request for consultation, if necessary), the anesthetist should discuss the proposed anesthesia plan with the patient. This discussion should include the risks and alternatives (see Informed Consent). It is imperative that all of the patient's questions be answered truthfully and that the patient accept the proposed plan. Documentation of preanesthesia evaluation is imperative. Many hospitals utilize a separate form for this purpose (Fig. 6-1). If these forms are not available, a note should be entered somewhere on the patient's chart concerning the preanesthesia evaluation.

Equipment

While modern technology has been instrumental in streamlining anesthesia practice, there is no question that depending entirely on mechanical devices carries inherent risks. Cooper lists seven steps to "safety and salvation" in his study.[10] He writes that one of the most frequently associated factors in anesthesia mishaps was unfamiliarity with the use of the equipment. A greater burden is placed on the anesthetist to acquire a sound theoretical and working knowledge of all anesthesia equipment; the anesthetist never be trapped into using new equipment without first obtaining adequate instruction.

Preventative maintenance of anesthesia equipment is an essential aspect of a risk management program. This should be performed and properly verified by a qualified technician.

Nerve Damage

Improper postioning of patients under anesthesia may lead to nerve damage and, invariably, a lawsuit. Assuming the responsibility for positioning patients in the OR is a prime example of "passing the buck." Surgeons want the patient placed in a position for surgical access, anesthetists are concerned about altered physiologic changes, and the OR nurse is often the person who actually positions the patient. Legal opinions have usually supported a shared responsibility in this respect. Proper charting is useful in showing exactly what happened and absolving one of liability.

The following case illustrates an example of a lawsuit resulting from nerve damage.

The patient brought medical malpractice action for injuries allegedly suffered by him during knee surgery. The plaintiff-patient, an excavation contractor, injured his knee while installing sewer pipe in a ditch when it caved in and buried him up to his waist. Rescuers extricated him from the ditch and transported him to a clinic where it was determined that his knee required surgery. The operation was scheduled for the following day.

DATE

TEMP PULSE RESP. BP.

DIAGNOSIS

HGB HCT. WT. HT.

SMOKING DRINKING

PROPOSED OPERATION

HISTORY

PHYSICAL EXAMINATION

INTUBATION ASSESSMENT
(AIRWAY, TEETH, NECK MOVEMENT)

RELEVANT LABORATORY FINDINGS

DRUG HISTORY	DOSE	DATES
STEROIDS		
HYPOTENSIVE		
INSULIN		
BETA-BLOCKER		
OTHER		
OTHER		
OTHER		

ALLERGY OR "HIVES" | IODINE PENICILLIN TAPE | "LOCAL" OTHER

BLEEDING TENDENCY

PREVIOUS ANESTHETICS

PREFER	ACCEPT	REJECT	SUMMARY AND PLAN
			LOCAL
			REGIONAL
			EPIDURAL
			SPINAL
			GENERAL

ASA 1 2 3 4 5
STATUS E

PRE-MED.

PRE-ANESTHETIC ATTENDING NOTE

SIGNED

M.D.

Fig. 6-1. Preanesthetic Assessment.

The patient suffered bilateral ulnar neuropathy after surgery and alleged that the cause was due to improper positioning on the operating table. The defendant surgeon and anesthesiologist argued that the plaintiff's ulnar nerve injury probably occurred during his extrication from the ditch and from improper handling during transportation to the clinic or during the postoperative period.

The defense verdict by the trial court was upheld on appeal on the basis that the plaintiff failed to establish by a preponderance of evidence that the injury was the kind that ordinarily did not occur in the absence of negligence. In other words, *res ipsa loquitur* did not apply.

Holmes v. Gamble, Col. App. 624 P.2d. 903 (1980)

REGIONAL ANESTHESIA

The selection of any anesthesia technique—regional, general, local, or conscious sedation—is determined by many factors, including surgical requirements, the patient's physical status, and the personal preference and habit of the anesthetist.

There currently is no statistical evidence that more lawsuits are filed following complications of regional anesthesia as compared to general anesthesia. The statistics do indicate, however, that there are more serious side effects from general anesthesia than from regional (spinal) techniques. In fact, an HEW insurance survey recommended, because many of the largest malpractice awards have been given for anesthesia accidents resulting in permanent brain damage, that hospital safety programs concerned with the administration of anesthesia should encourage local or spinal anesthesia when indicated.[12]

A Canadian survey of 78,746 patients who received spinal anesthesia in teaching hospitals in the 10-year period between 1959 and 1969 revealed no deaths attributable to spinal anesthesia. The cases studied indicated no permanent complications from the spinal and only two cases of neuropathy affecting lumbar segments and one case of abducens nerve paralysis.[13]

Although the fear of litigation should not be a major factor in the selection of regional as compared to general anesthesia, it is useful to consider some of the legal aspects that apply specifically to regional anesthesia.

Lawsuits arising from regional anesthesia generally relate to the known complications of these blocks. However, these complications and side effects, while unfortunate, are not necessarily indicative of negligence. Since the burden of proof in a negligence case is usually on the plaintiff, he or she must show that the complication was due to the act or omission of the defendant and that the care received was below the accepted standard of care (see Chapter 5).

Litigation arising from regional anesthesia blocks usually involves one or more of the following categories of legal action: lack of consent, negligence, or *res ipsa loquitur*.

Consent

Although the law of consent has been considered in a previous chapter, it is beneficial to deal with it again in relation to regional blocks. The current legal strategy of plaintiffs' attorneys is to claim lack of informed consent when there has been a complication following a regional block that results in a lawsuit (i.e., the plaintiff declares, "If I had known there was a chance that I could be paralyzed, I would not have agreed to the spinal").

Modern law on informed consent focuses on the informational needs of an average, reasonable patient, rather than on professionally established standards of disclosure. Under these rules, each anesthetist needs to develop a rapport with the patient, explain the type of block being considered, the risks and complications, as well as all possible alternatives. There is neither legal nor medical justification for attempting to hide the type of block from the patient by using terminology such as "nerve block" instead of "spinal anesthetic." The type of anesthestic must be explained in nontechnical terms that the patient can reasonably be expected to understand.

Most informed consent cases have arisen from the provider's failure to reveal sufficient information about the risks and consequences of the proposed regional anesthetic. A leading case in consent law, while not an anesthetic case, illustrates the importance of telling patients of potential complications.

In Canterbury v. Spence, a neurosurgeon failed to disclose to his 19-year-old patient that the lumbar laminectomy he was going to perform carried with it a risk of paralysis, estimated at trial by the physician-defendant to be about 1 percent. The patient did suffer paralysis, although it was never determined whether this was the result of the surgery or of a fall sustained during the immediate postoperative recovery period. The subsequent lawsuit alleged both negligent performance of the operation and failure to disclose a known risk.

In defense of his withholding the information the doctor testified: "I think that I always explain to patients the operations are serious, and I feel that any operation is serious. I think that I would not tell patients that they might be paralyzed because of the small percentage, 1 percent, that exists. There would be a tremendous percentage of people who would not have surgery and would not, therefore, be benefited by it, the tremendous percentage that get along very well, 99 percent."

The physician kept an important and highly sensitive piece of information from his patient, and by doing so, he violated the patient's right to self determination. The court, on appeal, held that the patient-plaintiff could maintain an informed consent suit even without producing expert testimony as to the professional community standard of disclosure in laminectomy cases.

Canterbury v. Spence, 150 U.S. App. D.C. 263, 464 F. 2d 772 (1972)

There have been a number of cases regarding lack of informed consent for regional anesthesia. In Beausoleiu v. Providential Sisters of Charity, a Canadian anesthetist convinced a patient that she should have a spinal after the patient had told the surgeon she did not want one. When she recovered from the anesthesia she was paralyzed from the waist down. The Canadian appellate court ruled: "Where there is no urgency, a doctor cannot submit a patient to risks the patient is unwilling to accept and if he does so and damage results, he is liable therefore and it is immaterial that the technique employed was above reproach or that what happened was a pure accident. . . . The administration of the spinal anesthetic was contrary to the express prohibition of the plaintiff and the fact that there was no malpractice in connection with the administration of anesthetic itself had no bearing on the liability of the doctor which was based on lack of consent."[14]

Negligence

The rules of negligence are the same in regional anesthesia litigation as with any type of malpractice case in that the plaintiff attempts to prove negligent activity and to collect damages. This burden of proof shifts to the defendent when the doctrine of *res ipsa loquitur* is applied. (see Chapter 5)

Since *res ipsa loquitur* literally means "the thing speaks for itself," it is obvious why this doctrine can be applied to a regional anesthesia case where a healthy patient is paralyzed or has other serious nerve damage after the anesthetic.

An example can be found in Senerio v. Haas, a 1961 California case:

> The patient, a 37-year-old mother of four was given a spinal anesthetic for a spontaneous and uncomplicated delivery. The next morning she complained that she could not move her legs—that she had pain in her back, neck, arms, and wrists. Within months she regained the use of her right leg, but at the time of the trial she still suffered pain in her left hip and had limited use of her left leg.
>
> The court ruling on application of *res ipsa loquitur* held that: "Where a plaintiff receives unusual injuries while in the course of medical treatment, all those defendants who had any control over her body, or the instrumentality which might have caused these injuries, may properly be called on to meet the inference of negligence by giving an explanation of their conduct."

Senerio v. Haas, 45 C 2d 811 P2d 911 (1950)

Complications from all types of regional blocks have led to legal action, but the greatest number in past years were from spinal administration. Some of the complications and reported litigation from the various regional blocks will assist the anesthetist in evaluating regional anesthesia practice.

Spinal Anesthesia

The complications from spinal blocks are categorized as either transient or permanent. The transient complications, such as headaches, backache, and abducens nerve palsy are annoying to the patient, but rarely result in a lawsuit. The permanent paralysis or nerve damage in an otherwise healthy patient, on the other hand, often leads to legal action. Anesthetists should be alerted to the state of the art techniques in prevention and treatment of side effects of spinals, including the use of fine-guage needles and techniques for treatment of postspinal headache.

The most serious deterrent to the use of spinal anesthesia is the possible occurrence of serious and permanent neurologic sequalae. When analyzing a neurologic deficit which develops after spinal anesthesia, Dornette advises a five-step approach.[15]

1. Determine the medical history of the patient with as much accuracy and completeness as possible, placing particular emphasis on the nervous system.
2. Assess the technique employed for the production of spinal anesthesia, including the equipment and sterilization of reusable equipment; special attention must be given to the occurrence of paresthesia during performance of lumbar puncture and administration of spinal anesthesia.
3. Determine whether there is a possibility that the operative technique may have produced or contributed to the neurologic defect.
4. Assess all aspects of the neurologic defect, including onset, extent of damage, progress or regression, and prognosis.
5. Determine whether the deficit is related causally to the anesthetic technique or other factors.

In reviewing legal cases involving spinal anesthesia, problems with technique and equipment, and inadequate preanesthesia evaluation, and monitoring of the patient can be found.

A patient developed an injury to the fifth lumbar and first sacral nerves on the left side after a spinal anesthetic. The defendant failed to prove that he repositioned the needle after the patient complained of excruciating pain on insertion. The verdict for the plaintiff was affirmed and the court noted: "It is significant that the anesthesiologist's anesthesia records are in error in some material respects and incomplete in others. This is a circumstance which we have considered in determining his adherence to the rules of his profession."

Herbert v. Travelers Indemnity Co., 221 So. 2d. LA (1969)

The following case was decided on lack of informed consent.

The facts in this case indicate that the plaintiff, John McKinney, consulted a surgeon regarding a large right inguinal hernia and a small left inguinal hernia. A spinal anesthetic was administered by an anesthesiologist. Following the operation, the patient suffered from permanent bilateral testicular atrophy, total sexual impotency, and numbness of the pubic and groin area. The patient sued the surgeon and anesthesiologist for damages. At the trial the expert witnesses reached several conclusions regarding the complications. They stated that the cause of the testicular atrophy was vascular damage at the time of surgery. It was suggested that the numbness was too extensive to be caused by the surgery and was most likely due to the spinal anesthetic.

Neither the surgeon nor the anesthesiologist had informed the patient of the risks of surgery or spinal anesthesia. The surgeon testified that he usually told his patients that there may be temporary swelling and numbness after a hernia operation; he claimed he told the patient only that it was a simple operation and there would be no problem. The plaintiff testified that had he been informed of the possibility of bleeding and testicular atrophy following the hernia operation or the possibility of losing sensation in his sexual organs he would not have consented to the operation.

A defense verdict for the anesthesiologist was upheld.

McKinney v. Nash, 120 Cal. App 3d 428 (1981)

In the following case, *res ipsa loquitur* was applied. The court found that due care was not exercised.

In 1959 the plaintiff, Arlene Mayor, was 34 years old and employed in the office of a contracting firm. She was also a vocalist and derived income from her singing. There was substantial evidence that she was in good health during her pregnancy and at the time of the birth of her child.

Mrs. Mayor was admitted to a Portland, Oregon hospital for delivery. At 9:48 A.M. on November 7, 1959, a resident physician administered a saddle block at the direction of the obstetrician. The saddle block injection was made at the L 4-5 interspace and consisted of novocaine 2.5 percent diluted in spinal fluid from the patient, making a total of 2 cc. At 9:52 A.M., the plaintiff gave birth to a normal baby boy.

The hospital record indicated that at 11:20 A.M., Mrs. Mayor complained of intermittent chilling. She was soon transferred to a private room, where she complained of shortness of breath. A nurse note at 12:30 P.M. read "blood pressure 104/80, patient rigid, and movement of arms spastic, nauseated." Shortness of breath and difficulty breathing were noted on the chart at 8:00 P.M. and again at 9:00 P.M.

At 7:15 A.M. the following morning, the patient suffered a convulsion and was completely unconscious. The hospital records indicate that respiration ceased at 8:30 A.M. and she was limp all over. A tracheostomy was performed and the tube was connected to a Bird respirator. At the time of the trial in June 1963, the patient was still partially paralyzed from the neck down and could breathe only with artificial aid.

There was expert testimony at the trial that there is evidence that the standard practice in Portland is to place a pillow under the patient's head after the spinal injection in order to guard against the danger of the anesthetic ascending the spinal canal. The patient testified that no pillow was used in her case.

There was evidence that permanent partial paralysis from the neck down is not expected to result from the delivery of a child following a spinal anesthetic when due care or proper practice are observed. The sole expert witness for the plaintiff was a general practitioner in Portland. He based his testimony on his experience, the history of the case, and the study of relevant medical literature. He testified that, in his opinion, Mrs. Mayor's paralysis was either directly or indirectly related to the administration of the anesthetic. On cross examination, he conceded that if the anesthetic reached the upper levels of the spinal canal, he would expect an immediate fall in blood pressure and embarassment of the patient's breathing.

The court found that use of *res ipsa loquitur* doctrine would apply.

Mayor v. Dawsett, 400 P. 2d. 234, Oregon

In the following case, the anesthesiologist was found negligent in the selection of an anesthetic.

An orthopedic procedure for the reduction of a trimalleolar fracture was prematurely terminated when the spinal anesthetic wore off. As a result of the premature closing, several loose bone fragments remained and the patient subsequently developed painful osteoarthritis. There was conflicting testimony whether the anesthesiologist had offered to supplement the disappearing anesthetic with meperdine or had concurred with the decision to close without affixing the posterior fragments.

The appellate court sustained the trial court's verdict against the orthopedic surgeon and the anesthesiologist. The court said that while the evidence was sufficient to show that there was not negligence in selecting a spinal rather than a general anesthetic, there was evidence that the anesthesiologist was negligent in selecting the agent to be used in the spinal (tetracaine 10 mg, without epinephrine). The orthopedic surgeon estimated the surgery would take from 2 to 3 hours to complete. The court also commented on the failure of the anesthesiologist to note the premature termination of the anesthetic in his anesthesia records, as he should have done. As a result, the court ruled that the jury could infer from such omission that he possessed some guilty knowledge concerning the termination.

Clark v. Gibbons, 58 Cal. Rptr 124 426 p 2d 525, (1967)

Monitoring of a spinal was an issue in a Massachusetts case where both the anesthesiologist and nurse anesthetist were named as codefendants.

The spinal was administered by the anesthesiologist who then turned the case over to a nurse anesthetist. Within the following 10 minutes, the nurse anesthetist could not get a blood pressure reading on the patient. She gave phenylephrine intramuscularly and then started an intravenous infusion. Because the patient had no heart beat, a thoracotomy and successful cardiac resuscitation followed. The patient's appendix was removed, but he never recovered consciousness and is essentially a neurologic vegetable.

The plaintiff alleged that spinal anesthesia was an improper choice because the patient had a history of rheumatic heart disease 12 years previously. The court held that any connection between the early attack and the patient's cardiac status at the time of the injury was pure conjecture.

Ramsland v. Shaw, 166 NW 2d 895 Mass. (1960)

Dornette, commenting on the Ramsland case, said that the facts suggest several departures from the standard of care, including failure to initiate an I.V. infusion before induction of the spinal anesthetic and turning the patient over to a nurse anesthetist before his condition had stabilized.[15]

Epidural Anesthesia

Neurologic damage, spinal headaches from inadvertent dural puncture, severed catheters, seizures from intravascular injection, and fetal depression are some of the complications arising from epidural blocks. A high percentage of epidurals are administered in obstetrics for labor and delivery, which explains why a number of the reported legal cases involving these blocks are obstetric cases.

"A 47-year-old male was admitted to a California hospital in 1979 for surgical repair of an ischiorectal abscess. The preanesthesia evaluation by the anesthesiologist revealed a 5'11", 250 lb. male in good health. His temperature was 38.4° C. The following premedication was given at 11:45 A.M.: morphine 12 mg and atropine 0.6 mg.

"An epidural block was administered at 12:20 P.M. with bupivacaine 0.5 percent in 28 cc. The patient was then placed prone on the operating table in a jacknife position. The systolic blood pressure dropped from 140 to 100 mm Hg and it remained about this level. There was no ECG monitor attached. The anesthesiologist monitored the radial pulse by palpation and spoke periodically with the patient. At 12:45 P.M., because of restlessness, Innovar® 1 cc was given with an additional 1 cc 5 minutes later.

"The patient settled down and then at 1:00 P.M., just at the close of surgery, his arms began to tremble violently and the radial pulse disappeared. There was some difficulty turning the patient, which took about 2 minutes, and endotracheal intubation was not accomplished for another 4 minutes. The patient was resuscitated, but died later that night.

"An autopsy revealed an enlarged liver—more than twice the normal size, with fatty infiltration. The coronary arteries were free of arteriosclerotic changes, but there was pronounced left ventricular enlargement.

"The negligence suit was settled out of court for a total of $180,000."

Alameda Superior Court No. 503680-3, reported in Rubsamen D: Professional Liability Newsletter, October 1979. Reprinted with permission.

In the following case, a negligence action was brought against one physician, hospital, and manufacturer of the anesthetic.

"A 35-year-old mother of seven children was admitted to a California hospital in June, 1973 for delivery. The pregnancy was at term and the cervix was 50 percent effaced. Buccal Pitocin® [oxytocin] was given. The obstetrician administered a caudal anesthetic consisting of Marcaine® [bupivacaine] 2 cc as a test dose, followed by 10 cc and 8 cc a short time later. Before each injection he aspirated on the plunger and observed no blood. The patient had no intravenous line established.

"Immediately after the third injection the patient began to seize. She had three seizures followed by a cardiac arrest. She was resuscitated but remained in a coma and died within 2 hours. Because of obvious fetal distress, an emergency cesarean section was performed.

"The baby was severely depressed. Although he has extremely severe cerebral palsy, he has a normal I.Q. His motor deficits involve all extremities, he can not hold up his head and has impaired function of his sphincters.

"There was a negligence action against the obstetrician, the hospital, and Winthrop Laboratories, manufacturers of Marcaine®. The hospital was named as a defendant because the obstetrician claimed that there was no crash cart in the room and that the emergency equipment was inadequate. He said there was no endotracheal equipment readily available. The obstetrician also indicated that there was too little help to deal with the emergency cesarean section. He also testified that he told the delivery room nurse to call a "code blue," but there was a delay of several minutes because she contacted her supervisor first.

Winthrop Laboratories was named in the suit for failure to provide information about the risk of convulsions from Marcaine®.

"The obstetrician settled out of court for $750,000 and the hospital settled for $350,000—for a total of $1,110.000. Winthrop took its case to a jury trial. Their defense rested on the fact that there is no increased risk of Marcaine® compared to other regional anesthetics, and that the drug information was adequate. The jury returned a verdict in favor of Winthrop."

Santa Barbara Superior Court No. SM 14774, reported in Rubsamen D: Professional Liability Newsletter, November 1978. Reprinted with permission.

Miscellaneous Blocks

Legal cases involving other anesthetic or therapeutic blocks are not as numerous as those from spinals and epidurals. This is perhaps because there is not the high incidence of neurologic and life-threatening complications. Cases reported include problems with the technique and lack of patient monitoring.

Brachial Block

The following case involves question of informed consent and negligence.

The patient had a brachial block anesthetic for surgery to remove a tumor from his right hand. The anesthesiologist, according to testimony, did not advise the patient of the complications inherent in the administration of the block, nor were possible alternatives suggested.

The plaintiff testified he felt two sharp pains when the anesthetic was administered and then lost consciousness. After the operation his shoulder was numb and after the numbness wore off, he had severe pain which lasted about 6 weeks. At the time of the trial, 3 years after the operation, he had not regained full use of his arm. The evidence established that the plaintiff suffered partial loss of the axillary nerve supply to the deltoid muscle which controls lifting of the arm from the shoulder.

The Oklahoma Appellate Court sustained defendant's demurrer to plaintiff's evidence. When applying the doctrine of informed consent to these facts the court said: "To establish liability under the 'informed consent' doctrine, an unrevealed risk must materialize, causing injury to the plaintiff and there must be a causal connection between failure to disclose and the injury. . . . A causal connection must exist between the physician's failure to disclose and the injury to the patient when disclosure of significant risks incidental to the treatment would have resulted in a decision by the patient against it."

Regarding the allegation of negligence, the court stated:

"Even though there was evidence that injection of a hypodermic needle into the brachial plexus of the patient's right shoulder to administer anesthesia could have caused patient's partial loss of axillary nerve supply to the shoulder muscle, where there were other occurrences which could have caused the injury, no evidence was introduced to exclude the other causes and there was no medical testimony to support finding that such injury from administration of brachial block was more likely the result of negligence than some other cause. Patient who brought action against physician did not establish that his injury was 'probably' caused by a thing under the exclusive control and management of the physician who administered the anesthetic for purposes of recovery under *res ipsa loquitur* doctrine."

Martin v. Stratton, 515 p 2d 1355 Oklahoma (1973)

The following case in another illustration of judicial interpretation of the need for informed consent.

The patient was admitted to the hospital for repair of a severe laceration of his right hand. He consented to a brachial block anesthetic which was administered by an anesthesiologist. During the procedure, the anesthesiologist punctured the patient's right lung, causing partial deflation. The pneumothorax was treated by a thoracic surgeon.

In a malpractice action against the orthopedic surgeon, the anesthesiologist, and the hospital, the patient claimed that the physicians failed to warn him of complications of a brachial block and that all three defendants (orthopedic surgeon, anesthesiologist, and thoractic surgeon) failed to provide proper postoperative care resulting in unnecessary pain for about 9½ hours while his lung was collapsing.

The Arkansas Supreme Court, in affirming the trial court's directed verdict against the patient, wrote that the patient failed to prove that the physician or hospital was negligent. Expert witnesses testified that it was impossible to tell how deep the brachial plexus and lung were below the surface because the thickness of the overlying soft tissue varied. The thoracic surgeon and anesthesiologist testified that there was no way to prevent an occasional lung puncture during the procedure.

The court said that there was no evidence that either physician was negligent nor was the hospital at fault for the nurses' failure to diagnose the patient's collapsed lung sooner.

Napier v. Northern, 572 S.W. 2d 153, Arkansas Supreme Court (1978)

PREVENTION AND DEFENSE OF LAWSUITS FROM REGIONAL ANESTHESIA

The decision to administer a regional anesthetic must be based on a combination of factors including the professional judgment of the anesthetist, preanesthesia status of the patient, and surgical needs. The selection of patients least likely to develop complications is of paramount importance when considering regional anesthesia from a legal perspective.

Preanesthesia Evaluation

It is particularly important for the anesthetist to ascertain any history of neurologic deficit or disease that may worsen or exacerbate after a regional anesthetic. Some authorities believe regional blocks are contraindicated in patients with any neurologic deficit, while others believe that if the disease is characterized by remissions and exacerbation a block may be given.[16]

Any other pre-existing condition that might lead to complications should also be carefully evaluated according to the type of block planned. Included are hypovolemia, anticoagulant therapy, and allergies to local anesthetic agents. The patient should also be carefully evaluated for any potential technical difficulties so that alternate techniques can be planned if necessary.

From the legal vantage, the preanesthesia evaluation must be properly recorded on the patient's chart and should include the fact that an informed consent was obtained.

Equipment and Supplies

A high proportion of lawsuits from spinals in previous years was due to complications from improper sterilization of equipment which led to infections and resulting neurologic deficits. The use of disposable equipment is encouraged, is probably cost effective, and lessens the chance of infection. If reusable trays are used, they must be properly sterilized and maintained and should be stored in such a manner that sterility is guaranteed.

Preparation of the OR equipment should be the same for a regional as for a general anesthetic. There have been numerous cases leading to lawsuits where a regional block was given without the patient having an I.V. line, with no means of positive pressure ventilation, and no readily accessible endotracheal equipment or resuscitative drugs. Most of these cases are settled out of court because of the difficulty in defending them and obtaining expert witnesses to attest to the standard of care.

Monitoring Patients

It is important that the nurse anesthetist does not assume a casual approach to monitoring patients under regional anesthesia.

Lawsuits stemming from inadequate monitoring, leaving the patient, or delay in recognizing complications would be very hard to defend.

Charts

Defense attorneys who specialize in medical malpractice cases often comment on the difficulty of defending a case when the charting has been poor. It appears that an anesthetist who usually charts adequately for general anesthesia cases, often is not as precise in charting regional anesthesia cases.

REFERENCES

1. London Medical Gazette 6:255, 1848
2. Althouse J: Rx:Loss Control—An analysis of anesthesia incidents: Part I. AANA J, February 1980, pp 59–60
3. Althouse J: Rx:Loss Control—An analysis of anesthesia related claims: Part II. AANA J, June 1980, pp 277–279
4. Minneapolis St. Paul Fire and Marine Insurance Co: Summary of anesthesia-related malpractice claims: Malpractice Digest May/June, 1980
5. Goldstein A, Keats A: The Risk of Anesthesia Anesthesiology, vol 33. 1970, pp 130–143
6. Taylor G, CP, Prestwick R: Unexpected cardiac arrest during anesthesia and surgery. JAMA 236 (24):2758–2760, 1976
7. Brunner E: Factors related to anesthetic risk. Surg Gynecol Obstet 141:761–762, 1975
8. Wylie WD: There, but for the grace of God. Annals of the Royal College of Surgeons of England. 56:171–180, 1975
9. Cooper J, Newbower R, Long C, McPeek B: Preventable anesthesia mishap: A study of human factors. Anesthesiology 49:399–406, 1978
10. Cooper J: Avoiding Preventable Mishaps. Chicago, ASA Refresher Course, 1979, p 235
11. U.S. Senate Subcommittee on Executive Reorganization: Medical Malpractice: The Patient Versus the Physician. Washington D.C., Government Printing Office, 1969, pp 3–4
12. U.S. Department of Health, Education, Welfare: Medical Malpractice. October 20, 1978
13. Noble AB, Muray JG: A review of the complications of spinal anes-

thesia with experience in Canadian teaching hospitals from 1959 to 1969. Can Anaesthesia Soc 18:1, January 1971
14. Beausoleiu v. Providential Sisters of Charity, 53 D.L.R. 2d 65 (Quebec Ct. Queen's Bench Appeal Side, 1964)
15. Dornette W: Legal Aspects of Anesthesia. Clinical Anesthesia Series 8:1,2 and 3. Philadelphia, Davis, 1972
16. Bromage P: Epidural Analgesia. Philadelphia, Saunders, 1978, p 707

7
Vicarious Liability

The responsibility or liability for negligent acts of a nurse anesthetist is a controversial area that is undergoing modification from both a legal and practice perspective. The controversy arises from the variety of employment situations under which nurse anesthetists practice, emerging legal recognition of nonliability of physicians for the actions of nurses, and changes in hospital liability laws.

AGENCY

Agency is the area of law which established the traditional legal concept that the master is responsible for the acts of the servant if they are performed within the scope of employment. The modern correlation is the agency relationship of employer-employee-independent contractor and the borrowed servant doctrine.

Employer-Employee

The doctrine of *respondeat superior,* translated literally means "let the master speak." Under this doctrine, the employer is liable for the negligent acts of an employee as long as the acts were committed within the scope of employment. The key point is whether an actual employer-employee relationship exists and whether or not the acts were within the scope of employment. Generally, an employer-employee relationship is established between parties when the employee, because of his employment, is entitled to benefits such as disability and unemployment insurance and has income taxes and social security taxes withheld from his salary.

Independent Contractor

An independent contractor relationship is established when a person performs work for someone, but acts as his own agent. The principal has no right of control over the manner in which the agent's work is performed. Since the independent contractor is generally responsible for his own actions, in cases of wrongful or negligent conduct the doctrine of *respondeat superior* does not apply. Nurse anesthetists, acting as independent contractors, would probably, therefore, be held legally reponsible for their actions. Recent court decisions have, however, established some degree of liability for hospitals for acts of their independent contractors because of the hospital's duty to be selective and responsible in evaluating the people they select to care for their patients.

Borrowed Servant

The "borrowed servant" theory is a special application of *respondeat superior* that may pertain to the situation when an employer loans an employee to another for a particular purpose. If a borrowed servant were working in a hospital OR, the "captain of the ship" concept would probably be accepted. The key being that the "captain" has the right to control and direct the actions of others. Some recent legal interpretations have modified the traditional approach to the "captain of the ship" doctrine, however (see below).

PHYSICIAN LIABILITY

The conventional approach to physician liability was often justified by the belief that a physician in ordering a nurse to perform a particular procedure would make a statement such as, "Don't argue, I take responsibility for all that you do." In light of recent court decisions, this approach is not only naive, but a legal delusion, if not a total fallacy.

Vicarious Liability

Physicians have believed in the "captain of the ship" doctrine which states that the surgeon is liable for all persons and activities in the OR that affect the patient. The origin of this doctrine can be traced to a Pennsylvania case, McConnell v. Williams (3 61 PA. 355 A. 2d 243 1943). In that case, a surgeon was controlling hemorrhage during a cesarean section. He turned the care of the newborn child over to an intern who was assisting him. The intern applied silver nitrate to the child's eyes. Apparently, as a result of the amount of solution applied, the infant suffered severe eye damage.

Although the surgeon in no way exercised control of the intern, the court held that he could be held vicariously liable in such a case. The test the court applied was whether other persons participating in the care of the patient were subject to the physician's control or right to control with regard to the work to be done and the manner of performing it. The court oserved that until the surgeon leaves the operating room "he is in the same complete charge of those who are present and assisting him as the captain of a ship over all on board."

Modern courts are recognizing the separation of responsibility among members of the surgical team as well as the specialized training needed to perform the different tasks. The trend is clearly moving away from the idea the the surgeon is the captain of the ship and, as such, liable for the negligence of others in the OR, particularly those over whom he does not have full control.

The California case that follows illustrates this trend.

A patient suffered severe brain damage caused by hypoxia from anesthesia administered by an anesthesiologist. In affirming a verdict for the surgeon, the court held that he (the surgeon) could not be held vicariously responsible for the actions of the anesthesiologist. The problems involving the patient's respiration were said to be within the jurisdiction of the anesthesiologist over whose performance the surgeon had no control or right to control.

Marvulli v. Elshire, 27 Cal. App 3d 180, 103 Cal. Rptr. 461 (1972)

The strongest case for relieving the surgeon of liability can be found in this New Jersey decision involving a nurse anesthetist.

The plaintiff was admitted to Muhlenberg Hospital for the delivery of her baby. The anesthesia was administered by a certified registered nurse anesthetist, an employee of the hospital. The hospital employed nurse anesthetists rather than anesthesiologists "since they were available 24 hours a day, and since the time of delivering babies could not be predicted or scheduled in advance."

The administration of the anesthetic involved the insertion of an airway into the patient's mouth. In addition to the airway, a catheter was inserted into her mouth through the airway and into her throat. The record contains facts and disputed inferences as to the actual manner in which plaintiff suffered her injury. In any event, it is clear that during the course of the delivery, she suffered damage to her teeth and mouth as a result of the administration of the anesthesia.

The court instructed the jury on the question of the hospital's liability as follows: "Defendant hospital admitted that. . . . the certified nurse anesthetist was employed by the hospital. Evidence indicates also that . . . (she) was assigned by the hospital to administer the anesthesia to Mrs. Sesselman in connection with the birth of her child. Under these circumstances, the hospital is legally responsible for any negligence of (the) nurse anesthetist."

The appeal court ruled on the vicarious liability of the obstetrician for the acts of the nurse anesthetist. They held that: "Nurse anesthetist, who was a hospital employee, did not become the legal servant or agent of the obstetrician merely because she received instructions from him as to the work to be performed during patient's childbirth; in absence of anything in the record to establish that, during the administration of the anesthetic and the dynamics of the birth, obstetrician undertook to exercise control over the nurse's activities, obstetrician was not removed from the general rule of nonliability."

Sesselman V. Muhlenberg Hospital, 124 NJ Super. 285 (1973)

In summary, it appears that, with few exceptions, the law is moving to remove any vicarious liability from surgeons for the negligent acts of trained personnel who are working with them—so long as surgeons do not exercise control over those persons or stand in the active position of being their employer.[1]

HOSPITAL LIABILITY

The liability of a hospital for anesthetic injury is usually based on the laws of *respondeat superior* where the hospital assumes the responsibility for its employees. In relatively recent legal decisions, hospital liability has been expanded to include acts of independent contractors and others who use the hospital facilities. Whether a hospital will actually be judged liable under *respondeat superior* for the negligence of anesthetists depends, of course, on the circumstances of each case as they affect the questions of agency and the elements of actionable negligence.[2]

The hospital, as a corporation entity, may also be found liable in anesthesia cases for failure to provide and maintain proper equipment, sufficient, well-trained personnel, adequate safety precautions, and skilled postanesthesia recovery teams.

LIABILITY FOR ACTS OF ANESTHESIA

A hospital's liability for the negligent acts of an employee under the agency doctrine of *respondeat superior* is upheld in a number of cases involving anesthetists or anesthesiologists.[3-5] The test of hospital liability is whether the acts committed were performed in the service of the hospital and whether the acts were within the scope and course of the employee's duties. The courts, in past years, generally have not held hospitals liable for anesthesia mishaps when the anesthesia was administered by an independent contractor.

The court rejected a patient's contention that a hospital was responsible for a spinal anesthetic injury on the theory of agency. The patient had been admitted to the hospital for a hemorrhoidectomy. The anesthetic was to be administered by an anesthesiologist who was a partner in "Anesthesia Associates." When the anesthesiologist inserted the needle into the patient's spinal canal, the patient gave out a cry of intense pain and complained that his left leg felt like it had been subjected to a severe electrical shock. Following the operation, which the patient acknowledged to have been completely satisfactory, the patient continued to experience pain in his left leg and foot. He received 150 physiotherapy treatments and then brought suit for damages against the anesthesiologist, Anesthesia Associates, their insurer, two surgeons, and the hospital. He alleged that the hospital was liable because the anesthesiologist, a physician, "did all of his work at the hospital, under the rules of the hospital."

In rejecting this contention, the court said that the record failed to disclose any legal basis whatsoever for the plaintiff's suit against the hospital. If there was any fault or negligence in the adminstration of the spinal anesthetic, said the court, it was that the anesthesiologist who, as an independent specialist, was wholly responsible for the instruments used, the method employed, and the professional judgment, technique and skill applied.

Herbert v. Travelers Indemnity Co., 193 So 2d 330 LA (1966)

The trend against hospital liability for independent contractors has now been reversed in many cases. In a case involving an emergency room physician, the appellate court said that even if the doctor was an independent contractor, the hospital held itself out to the public as providing facilities and appropriate staff, including doctors, for emergency treatment. Patients, the court held, could not be bound by secret limitations in a private contract between the hospital and the physician.[6]

The landmark decision that changed the relationship between doctors and hospitals was Darling v. Charleston Community Hospital.[7] In the case, the court recognized that a hospital could be liable for the acts and omissions of independent contractors. In several side issues, the Darling case addressed the problem of a hospital's legal obligation to ensure the quality of medical care within its walls. The Darling case also established that a hospital's own bylaws could be admitted in evidence, even if they are more rigorous than the local community standards. The court also allowed the admission in evidence of the standards of the JCAH because the hospital's bylaws reflected those guidelines.

More recent cases stress the duty of the hospital to insure that the staff and any others who use the facilities are carefully selected and evaluated.

A patient had received an injury to his eye that required surgery. The anesthesia was negligently administered and the patient suffered severe brain damage following a cardiac arrest. Other anesthesiologists, surgeons, and nurses at the hospital knew that the anesthesiologist was a drug user. The hospital and its director of anesthesia were on notice about possible danger to patients because they knew of several episodes in which the anesthesiologist was under the influence of drugs, as he was during the surgery that triggered the suit. The jury awarded the plaintiff $834,790.

Eng v. Valley Memorial Hospital, No. 460898-3 Oakland Sup Ct Cal (1978)

This Washington case is an example of a hospital's negligence in relation to a violation of its own rules.

The plaintiff was injured in an automobile accident and admitted to the hospital under the care of a physician. After treatment of minor injuries, it was determined that the patient had suffered a fractured jaw. A dentist was employed to repair the fracture. The anesthesia was adminis-

Vicarious Liability

tered by a nurse anesthetist employed by the hospital. The dentist testified that he had no working knowledge of the use or administration of a general anesthetic and the he had left the responsibility and control of the anesthesia procedure to the nurse anesthetist. There was no medical doctor present in the OR.

The patient suffered a convulsive seizure in the recovery room. The admitting physician could not be located and there was no other medical doctor available in the hospital at the time. Later, after a physician was found, the decision was made to transfer the patient to a large hospital in Seattle. He remained unconscious for over a month and there was evidence of permanent brain damage.

The nurse anesthetist testified that she had been a narcotic user for about 2 years and had recently replaced her drug addiction with the use of alcohol. At the trial, she had a minimum of independent recollection of the case and relied almost entirely on the anesthesia chart to describe what had transpired in surgery. She was hired and paid by the hospital who then billed the patient for her services.

The hospital had as one of its rules that "patients requiring dental service may be co-admitted by a member of the medical staff and a local dentist who is qualified, legally, professionally, and ethically to practice here. The former shall perform an adequate medical examination prior to any dental surgery, and be responsible for the patient's medical care."

In its holding on the case, the Washington Supreme Court ruled that it was negligent, as a matter of law, for a hospital to permit a surgical operation upon a patient under general anesthetic, in the absence of extraordinary or emergency circumstances, without the presence and supervision of a medical doctor in the OR. The court also held that in this particular case the hospital's negligence was underscored by the violation of its own rules. . . .

Penderson v. Dumouchel, 72 Wash 2d 73,431 P 2d 973, 31 ALR 3d 1100 (1967)

Because the laws affecting legal liability may be unfamiliar, nurse anesthetists are advised to review current JCAH standards and/or state laws regarding administration of anesthesia for dentists.

NURSE ANESTHETIST LIABILITY

Nurse anesthesia is clearly a profession in which each member assumes liability and responsibility for his or her individual acts. Courts are reversing their traditional rules whereby physicians are considered liable for a nurse's acts and are now generally holding the nurse or nurse's employer liable for the negligent acts or omissions. As nurses in general are being called upon to exercise independent judgment in many situations, legal accountability is implied. Practicing nurse anesthetists need to assess their employment status to determine where they stand in regard to malpractice insurance coverage. Free-lance anesthetists, who practice as independent contractors or who are in other types of private practice situations, must carry their own insurance or verify coverage by the hospital or other employer, if so agreed to in a contract.

Anesthetists employed by a hospital, clinic, professional or business corporation, or any other employer-employee relationship, should ascertain the existence of malpractice insurance and be cognizant of the limits of liability of the employer. It would be foolish for any anesthetist to practice without insurance or without clarification, preferably in writing, as to the the terms of professional liability insurance carried by the employer. It must never be assumed that physicians, whether surgeons or anesthesiologists, will take the liability and legal responsibility for the professional acts of a nurse anesthetist upon themselves.

PROFESSIONAL LIABILITY INSURANCE

Insurance is a contract in which the insurer agrees to assume certain risks of the insured in return for consideration or payment of a premium. Policy holders should recognize the components of the insurance policy and the rights, duties, and limitations of the policy. Although there are variations between insurance companies, standard liability coverage usually contains five distinct parts: insurance agreement, defenses and settlement, policy period, amount payable, and conditions.

Agreement

Agreement pertains to the terms of the policy in which it is stated what defined risks the company will assume for what precise amount of premium. It also indicates that the insurer has no obligation to pay any sum over and above the legal liability.

Defenses and Settlement

Defenses and settlements is an agreement between the insured and the insurance company that the company will defend any lawsuits against the insured arising from performance or nonperformance of professional duties. The company is also delegated the power to effect a settlement of any claims as it deems necessary, usually with the consent of the insured.

Policy Period

The period of the policy is always stated in the body of the insurance contract. Any accident that occurs before the policy is in effect or after the policy period would not be covered by the insurance agreement.

Claims

Many policies provide coverage for only those claims instituted during the policy period, while *occurrance* types of policies provide coverage for all claims that may arise out of the policy period.

Amount Payable

The amount to be paid by the insurer is determined by the amount of damages suffered by the injured party. This amount may be determined by a jury, judge, or an out-of-court settlement between the parties. The insurance company will pay no more than the maximum amount of coverage that is stated in the policy. The cost of any damage award over and above the policy limits will be borne by the insured.

Conditions of the Policy

Each insurance policy contains a number of conditions. Failure to comply with these conditions could result in forfeiture and nonpayment of claims. The following conditions generally are found:

1. Notice of occurance. Oral or written notification must be made by the insured to the insurance company of any injury that has occurred as a result of acts covered by the policy.

2. Notice of claim. When the insured receives notice that a claim or suit is being instituted, he or she must notify the insurance company immediately.
3. Assistance of the insured. The insured must cooperate with the insurance company and render any assistantce necessary to defend the claim or to reach a settlement.
4. Cancellation. The cancellation clause spells out the conditions and procedures necessary for either party to cancel the policy.

REFERENCES

1. Isele W: Vicarious liability in the operating room. Legal Med, April, 1975
2. Hospital Liability for Anesthetic Injuries. 31 ALR 3d 1114 2(a)
3. Calvero v. Franklin General Benev. Soc., 36 Cal. 2d 301, 222 P 2d 471 (1950)
4. Quintal v. Laurel Groves Hospital, 62 Cal. 2d 154, 41 Cal. Rptr. 577, 397 P 2d 161 (1964)
5. Lathon v. Hadley Memorial Hospital, Dist. Col. App. 250 A 2d 548 (1969)
6. Meduba v. Benedictus Hospital, 384 N.Y.S. 2d 527 (1976)
7. Darling v. Charleston Community Memorial Hospital, 33 111. 2d 326, 211 N.E. 2d 353 (1965)

8
Employment Law

Nurse anesthesia is a unique profession because of the variety of employment situations it entails. Salaried postions may exist where the employer is a hospital, a professional corporation of physicians and/or anesthetists, a university, or a Federal or State government. There are also private practices where the nurse anesthetist, as an individual or a corporation, contracts with a facility for anesthesia services or works temporarily on a freelance basis.

Some of the legal ramifications of the various types of practice were covered in the chapter on vicarious liability. There are many other situations where knowledge of the laws would be useful to the nurse anesthetist, such as circumstances pertaining to civil rights, laws on hiring practices, legalities of labor unions, contract law, and incorporation.

The laws are changing rapidly in many of these areas, and any presentation of them can only serve as a general overview of the subject. Nurse anesthetists are beginning to assert their legal rights in many of these employment fields, which should verify the status of the profession and serve as a model for other members of the profession. In fact, an important antitrust action was just filed this year by a nurse anesthetist against a number of hospitals and organizations for denial of clinical privileges.

CIVIL RIGHTS

The United States Constitutuion, along with acts of congress and state legislatures, guarantees certain rights to the people. Congress passed the Civil Rights Act in 1964, which included the Fair Employment Practice Act, known as Title VII. The essence of Title VII is the prohibition of discrimination on the basis of race, color, religion, sex, or national origin by employers, unions, or employment agencies. The provisions of this law apply to employers engaged in any industry affecting commerce and employing more than 15 people.

Legislation passed in 1978 expressly prohibited employers covered by Title VII from discriminating with respect to employment opportunities on the basis of pregnancy, childbirth, or related conditions. The federal legislation embodied in Title VII applies to all aspects of employment—hiring, salary, firing, benefits, and any other conditions of employment.

The Equal Pay Act was enacted in 1963 as an amendment to Section 6 of the Fair Labor Standards Act. This law makes it illegal for an employer to pay wages "at a rate less than the rate he pays employees of the opposite sex in such establishments for equal work on the job, the performance of which reqires equal skill, effort, and responsibility, and which are performed under similar working conditions."[1] The act was tested in hospital situations where courts generally have ruled that the work of female nursing aides and male orderlies be made "equal" under the Act, since the additional duties, responsibilities, or lifting of weight was not substantial.[2]

Practical Aspects

As employees, nurse anesthetists need to have an awareness of the civil rights laws that have impact on their individual work situations. Employers generally have developed personnel policies that require adherence to the various employment civil rights laws. These include hiring practices, orientation, evaluation, employee development, corrective action, and dismissal. Policies should be stated in writing and available to employees. If there is a suspected violation of these laws by an employer, employees should exercise their rights and seek the appropriate remedy.

The following is an example of policies and procedures that reflect civil rights laws.

Employment Practices—A model of rules and Regulations

General. It is the policy of the institution to initiate comprehensive written affirmative action personnel policies to provide applicants and employees with the right to equal employment opportunity. The institution will not engage in discriminatory practices against any person because of race, color, religion, marital status, national origin, sex, age, or citizenship.

Hiring. Selection of employees involves indentifying and hiring the most qualified applicant for a particular position. The process requires that each position be clearly defined and the knowledge, skills, and other qualifications required be accurately stated.

Orientation. After an employee is appointed to a position, it is the supervisor's responsibility to see that a proper orientation is accomplished. Specifically, an employee needs to know about employee rights and responsibilities under the appropriate policies and procedures, the goals of the work unit, and the tasks for which the employee will be held responsible.

Evaluation. The employee must be informed of the standards that will be used to assess his or her work. A formal and an informal assessment or evaluation of job performance will be made on a regular basis.

A formal appraisal process requires analysis and evaluation of the employee's work performance and accomplishments. It also should include the setting of goals for future efforts, performance related strengths and weaknesses, and identification of problems.

Corrective Action. Whenever an employee fails to meet the required standards of conduct or performance, necessary and appropriate corrective action will be initiated. Corrective action ranges from written warnings to suspension without pay. When taking corrective action, it is necessary to identify and discuss with the employee particular performance problems and develop an explicit plan for improvement.

Dismissal. Dismissal, except for certain well-defined reasons, is normally made only after corrective action has been unsuccessful. Specific procedures should be described to assure fair and equitable treatment of all employees.

The dismissal of a nurse anesthetist who asserted her "right of conscience" was overturned by an appellate court in the following case.

A nurse anesthetist advised the administration of the hospital where she worked that she would not participate in a tubal ligation. Her objection was based on moral and religious grounds. Since there was such a procedure scheduled for the next day, the administrator obtained the services of another nurse anesthetist from a hospital 50 miles away.

When she was advised verbally that she was fired, the nurse anesthetist requested a written statement containing the reasons for her dismissal. The administrator wrote: "Your untimely refusal to perform customary and needed services puts me in a position where I have few viable alternatives." No request was made by the hospital or the person desiring the sterilization that the anesthetist state, in writing, her grounds for refusing to participate.

Montana, the state where the incident happened, has a statute that states that a person's refusal to participate in sterilization, when based upon religious beliefs and moral convictions, shall not be a consideration in respect to staff privileges nor a basis for any disciplinary or discriminatory action. The trial court ruled that the employer's necessities outweighed the anesthetist's rights under the Conscience Statute.

The appellate court overturned this ruling and concluded that the refusal of the anesthetist to participate in the sterilization was timely. The court took particular notice of the fact that the sterilization was an elective procedure in this case and that there was nothing to show that the hospital was unduly prejudiced or that the patient was in danger.

Swanson v. St. John's Lutheran Hospital, 597 P. 2d 702 (1980)

CONTRACT LAW

In an increasing number of employment situations, nurse anesthetists are entering into a contractual relationship with an employer. The importance of understanding the basic elements of contract law, therefore, cannot be overemphasized. As in all legal considerations, it is advisable to seek the services of a competent, knowledgeable attorney when drafting an employment contract.

A *contract* is defined as a promissory agreement between two or more parties, that creates, modifies, or destroys a legal relationship. Any valid contract, whether an employment contract or one for other purposes, contains certain elements: mutual assent, promise or consideration, two or more parties who have legal capacity, and a lawful purpose that is not against public policy.

Mutual assent simply means that there is a clear understanding between all parties. There must be both an offer and an acceptance in clear, definite, and communicated terms. The objective expressed intention of the offeror and offeree determines if a contract is created.

Consideration refers to whatever is given in exchange for something else. The essential criteria is that the parties have bargained with one another and have exchanged a promise for a promise or a promise for the performance or nonperformance of an act.

In order for a contract to be valid, it must be entered into by parties who are mentally competent, who are in full possession of their faculties and not under any legal disability or duress. Persons who by reason of insanity, who are under the influence of alcohol or drugs, or who have not reached the age of majority generally are considered incompetent to make a contract. Contracts that are illegal or against public policy are not enforceable.

Breach of Contract

Because the courts recognize legally enforceable contracts, there are certain legal remedies available if a contract is breached. Breach of contract is the unjustified failure to perform according to the terms of a contract that was agreed upon or to act when performance is due. The remedies available for such a breach are money damages, specific performance, or an injuction. Any one of the remedies, a combination of them, or all of them may be awarded.

Damage awards for breach of contract generally are limited to what the defendant could reasonably foresee at the time of making the contract would probably be the result of such breach. Specific performance may be sought when money damages would not be a satisfactory remedy. This would be a situation where the promise or act agreed upon was a special or unique type of performance. The third remedy for breach of contract, an injunction, is a special court order to stop a party to the contract from performing the specific promise or act under other circumstances.

Table 8-1
Elements to be included in Contracts between Nurse Anesthetists and Their Employers

Hospital and Staff Nurse Anesthetist	*Hospital and Group Practice of which Nurse Anesthetist Is an Employee*
Parties and date of agreement Identification of parties involved and intent of the agreement Scope of agreement 1. Employment 2. Services 3. Term 4. Compensation 5. Vacation and sick leave 6. Educational leave 7. Health and disability insurance 8. Miscellaneous benefits 9. Facilities 10. Malpractice insurance 11. Mutual assent	Parties and date of agreement Identification of parties Scope of agreement 1. Exclusive employment agreement 2. Services that group agrees to perform 3. Working hours-coverage 4. Qualifications of members of the group 5. Charges 6. Benefits group is entitled to, if any 7. Liability insurance 8. Medical record confidentiality 9. Disclaimer concerning hospital's responsibility for the professional judgment of the group 10. Services the employing institution agrees to perform for the group 11. Terms of agreement 12. Termination clause 13. Mutual assent

Classification of Contracts

Contracts are classified as either express or implied. Express contracts are those in which the terms have been agreed upon between the offeror and the offeree orally or in writing. Implied contracts give rise to contractual obligations through other legal mechanisms. An oral contract, when all the necessary elements are present, is binding. A written contract, however, is easier to enforce because a document can be produced in which the terms are clearly stated.

Employment Law

Table 8-1 (continued)

Group Practice and a Nurse Anesthetist Employee	*Independent Contractor and Hospital, Clinic, etc.*
Parties involved and date of agreement Identification of parties involved Scope of agreement 1. Employment 2. Services 3. Term 4. Termination clause 5. Compensation 6. Vacation and sick leave 7. Educational leave 8. Health and disability insurance 9. Facilities provided by the group 10. Malpractice insurance 11. Travel expenses 12. Mutual assent	Parties and date of agreement Identification of parties involved Scope of agreement 1. Qualifications of employee 2. Professional services provided 3. Adminstrative relationship 4. Working hours 5. Billing privileges 6. Disclaimer concerning responsibility of institution for nurse anesthetist's actions 7. Malpractice insurance 8. Services institution will provide nurse anesthetist 9. Compliance with laws, rules, and regulations 10. Term 11. Termination clause 12. Mutual assent

Employment Contracts

It may be advisable for a nurse anesthetist to consider the advantages of an employment contract as a means of job protection and a way to provide a clear understanding of the terms and scope of employment. The contract may be as simple as a letter from a hospital administratior spelling out the terms of employment or it can be a formally drawn-up legal document.

Samples of various contracts that can be adapted to nurse anesthetist employment are contained in the appendix. Up-to-date information and sample contracts may also be obtained from the Legislative-Employment Practices Coordinator, American Association of Nurse Anesthetists, 216 Higgins Road, Park Ridge, Illinois.

An employment contract will probaby contain different sections depending upon the scope of the agreement. Table 8-1 is a listing of minimum areas that should be included in contracts between nurse anesthetists and various types of employers (for sample contracts see Appendixes beginning on p 130).

Exclusive Contract

An area of employment contract law that has become increasingly controversial is in regard to exclusive contracts for hospital-based services such as anesthesia. Such an arrangement excludes any one who is not party to the agreement from practicing those services in the institution. A number of legal challenges have been made by physicians who claim an offense to professional pride, a denial of economic opportunity, and an interference in the patient-physician relationship.[3] Some of the exclusive contracts have been upheld because the courts have determined that they do have have the authority to review the decisions of private hospitals regarding exclusive agreements.[3]

Several court cases illustrate judicial support of exclusive contracts.

In Hughes v. J. Jefferson Parish Hospital, No. 78–750, E.b. 1/20/81, the court refused to find that the hospital's arrangement with a group to provide anesthesia services was in violation of antitrust laws, equal protection, and due process. These theories had been advanced by a non-group anesthesiologist who had been denied appointment to the hospital staff by virtue of the exclusive arrangement.

In Capili v. Mott, 620 F. 2d 438 4th Cir. (1980), a federal court of appeals upheld the exclusive anesthesia arrangements on the basis that it was justified by the hospital's and the community's needs. The hospital involved had a history of attemping to assure on-call services of anesthesiologists and nurse anesthetists, but had been dissatisfied when such services were not readily available. In addition, the JCAH had cited the hospital for a number of deficiencies in its provision of anesthesia service. Because of these problems and because the hospital believed that it had the burden of responsibility to assure the proper quality and quantity of anesthesia service to its patients, the hospital entered into an exclusive arrangement to insure the availablity of 24-hour-a-day, 7-days-a-week coverage by physician and nurse anesthetist services.

The court found that the arrangement was reasonably related to assuring the availability of anesthesia services to the hospital's patients, and that it also permitted efficient surgery, promoted the uniform selection and use of anesthesia equipment, and permitted centralized control of the responsibility for the rendering of service.

Although these cases illustrate court decisions which upheld exclusive contracts, provided they were justified on the grounds of patient care and hospital responsibility, the antitrust and civil rights implications continue to be challenged.

The advantages of a written contract over an oral one is illustrated in this nurse anesthetist case.

In a contractual dispute between five nurse anesthetists and Woman's Hospital of Baton Rouge, Louisiana, an oral termination agreement was upheld. When the hospital began operation in 1968, four C.R.N.A.s began providing professional services at the request of the founding physicians. They were entirely responsible for providing obstetric anesthesia; they made their own schedules; billed their patients individually; and provided their services on a 24-hour-a-day, year-round basis. The quality of their work and their efficiency was well known and respected by the physicians who practiced with them. Unfortunately, these C.R.N.A.s had no *written contractual agreement* with the hospital. The verbal agreement worked well until April, 1977, when the hospital administrator advised them that effective May, 1977 all C.R.N.A.s administering anesthesia would have to be in the employment of a newly engaged medical anesthesiologist. None of the nurse anesthetists accepted this arrangement.

The medical staff believed the change was necessary because of new developments in anesthesia and because the C.R.N.A.s were limited in the type of anesthesia they could administer, and that obstetric anesthesia should be under the complete control of a physician anesthesiologist.

The C.R.N.A.s terminated their services on May 1, 1977. Thereafter they sued the hospital, asserting breach of contract under which there was an agreement for 6 months notice before termination of their working agreement with the hospital. The District Court granted judgment to the plaintiff nurse anesthetists and the hospital appealed. The Court of Appeals of Louisiana, affirmed the judgment of the trial court in favor of the nurse anesthetists. They held that (1) the trial court correctly found that the hospital had effectively guaranteed the nurses 6 months notice, (2) there had been discussions concerning a written contract, in lieu of which, the oral promise to provide 6 months notice was enforceable against the hospital, (3) the 6 month notice of termination was not given by the hospital, and (4) the nurses made a reasonable effort to minimize the damages.

The appellate court evaluated cumulative evidence of minutes of meetings of the Board of Directors of the hospital. These records, taken together with undisputed allegations by the nurse anesthetists that they had individually signed an agreement, which later proved to have been a recommendation from the Ad Hoc Anesthesia Committee to the Board of Directors, constituted sufficient evidence of the parties.

Herbert v. Woman's Hospital Foundation, 377 So 2d 1340 La. (1980)

LABOR LAW

Labor law is essentially a body of statutory laws based primarily upon federal labor statutes. The great bulk of the reported cases in labor law is the product of decisions by the National Labor Relations Board (NLRB) and their review by the federal courts of appeal and the United States Supreme Court. The NLRB is the federal administrative agency that administers the National Labor Relations Act.

Historically, the labor movement has its roots in the "sweat shops" of the late 18th and early 19th centuries. But it was not until 1935 that the National Labor Relations Act gave employees the right to form, join, or assist labor oranizations to bargain collectively through representatives of their own choosing and to engage in other activities for the purpose of collective bargaining, mutual aid, or protection.

The Taft-Hartley Amendments to the National Labor Relations Act in 1947 specifically excluded nonprofit hospitals, taking away the rights of those employees to organize. Employees in proprietary hospitals retained the right to organize. In 1974, the National Labor Relations Act was amended to again extend collective bargaining rights to employees of health care institutions, and nonprofit hospitals.

The right of unions to organize and the rights of employees and employers under the labor laws are a complex subject that is not within the scope of this book. The topic of collective bargaining, however, presented some interesting considerations for nurse anesthetists in employment situations where unions are active.

Provisions for collective bargaining are provided in the National Labor Relations Act, Section 8 (a)(5) which states that it is an unfair labor practice for an employer "to refuse to bargain collectively with the representatives of his employees, subject to the provisions of Section 9 (a)." The provisions of 9 (a) state that a bargaining representative of the employees shall be: (1) selected by a majority of the employees, (2) in an appropriate unit, (3) the *exclusive* representative of *all* the employees in that unit, and (4) for the purpose of collective bargaining in respect to rates of pay, wages, hours of employment, or other conditions of employment.

A major issue for many nurse anesthetists is the question of what constitutes a bargaining unit in a hospital and where they fit in. There have been several court rulings on this question with differing opinions from some jurisdictions.

In Wing Memorial Hospital Association and Massachusetts Nurses' Association v. The NLRB, 217 NLRB 172 (1975), it was determined that all registered nurses employed by the hospital in Palmer, Massachusetts, including the diabetic teaching nurse, the admissions coordinator, the *nurse anesthetist,* charge nurses, and head nurses, but excluding all other employees and supervisors, constituted an appropriate unit for the purpose of collective bargaining.

In a Minnesota case, petitions for the Minnesota Foundation of Certified Nurse Anesthetists to be recognized as a separate bargaining group were denied.[4] In the opinion from the NLRB, it was concluded: . . . "units limited to nurse anesthetists are inappropriate for the purposes of collective bargaining. In reaching this conclusion . . . [reliance is placed] on the facts that nurse anesthetists are registered nurses and hold identical statutory licenses; that registered nurses can and do pursue the numerous specialties in the profession; that nurse anesthetists reflect merely a specialty which a registered nurse may cultivate and achieve within the nursing profession; that the nurses' duties and objectives, be they specialized and limited or in the broad health care application, are to provide professional care; that the nurse anesthetists engage in substantial professional intercourse in that they spend a significant amount of time rendering direct patient care in association and in conjuction with other registered nurses; and that nurse anesthetists share common benefits and working conditions. Finally, a contrary conclusion would proliferate bargaining units and fragment collective bargaining within the health care institutions in violation of the Congressional and Board directives."

National Labor Relations Board Case No. 18 RC 12148 (1979)

A different result was obtained in Washington where the Group Health C.R.N.A. Employees Group was permitted to be an appropriate bargaining unit. In the NLRB decision it was stated:

" . . . Nurse anesthetists are supervised by the head of the anesthesiology department, whereas the registered nurses in the other sections of the hospital and employer's operation are supervised by the head of the department of nursing. There is some contact between the nurse anesthetists and the other registered nurses at the employer's operation along with other hospital employees as is necessary in providing health care to individual patients. Other registered nurses and employees cannot perform the duties of a nurse anesthetist, and there is no interchange between nurse anesthetists and registered nurses. . . .

"I find that the unit requested by the Petitioner C.R.N.A. is appropriate in light of the facts that formal and informal bargaining between the C.R.N.A. and the employer has existed for over 10 years . . . , the duties and responsibilities of the nurse anesthetist and registered nurse are substantially dissimilar, the lack of interchange betweem registered nurses and nurse anesthetists, and the separate supervision of the nurse anesthetists. . . ."

Group Health Cooperative of Puget Sound v. Group Health C.R.N.A. Employees Group, NLRB 19–UC–126. 18 RC–7314 (1975)

Once a collective bargaining unit has been established its primary purpose is to negotiate a union contract between the hospital and the union members. The basic structure of a union for nurses is found in the appendix. An excellent book, *Nurse Power, Union and the Law* by Karen O'Rourke and Sally Barton (Bowie Maryland 1981, Robert J. Brady Co.), gives a very comprehensive picture of labor unions for nurses.

The subject of unionization for professionals is an emotional one that has become complicated by conflicting court rulings. Any nurse anesthetist or group of anesthetists should become knowledgeable on all the ramifications, legal, professional, and personal, before committing themselves to joining a union. There is no question that unionization has been the only effective route for some nurse anesthetists in obtaining fair treatment from employers. Other nurse anesthetists have found it unacceptable to be placed in bargaining units with non-nurse anesthetists or, even worse, non-professionals.

Whatever route is taken, it is absolutely essential that the individuals who undertake to negotiate employment contracts for nurse anesthetists, whether union or non-union, have an understanding of the uniqueness of nurse anesthesia practice and hold the best interests of the profession as a number-one priority.

REFERENCES

1. Garland v. California Society of Anesthesiologists et al., United States District Court, Northern District of California. #C814278 (1981)
2. Hodgson v. Golden Isles Nursing Home, CA 5–1972, 9 FEP, Cases 791
3. Kucera W: The courts look at exclusive contracts for providing anesthesia services. JAANA April, 1981
4. Minnesota Federation of Certified Anesthetistis, et al. NLRB Case No. 18 RC 12148, etc. (1979)

9
Anesthesia—Legal Cases

The cases in this chapter are presented to give the nurse anesthetist an overview of the legal climate concerning medical malpractice as it presently exists. Avoiding a malpractice suit is, naturally, a prime consideration. However, being knowledgeable about the anatomy of a lawsuit, the critical areas of testimony and admissible evidence, and the rights and responsibilities of the parties concerned can be invaluable in the event of involvement in such legal action. A lawsuit, obvbiously, becomes easier to defend when the defendants have at least some knowledge in these areas.

The reader will quickly note that the facts relating to the anesthesia management of the cases presented are sparse and in some cases lead to more questions than answers. While this is frustrating at times, it is still apparent that even with limited facts, the anesthestist can obtain valuable information from these cases. By comparing what happened in a given case with his or her clinical practice, an anesthetist may be able to identify areas that need improvement or monitoring.

The judgments given and damages awarded should alert nurse anesthetists to their areas of responsibility and their legal liability in the event of a malpractice action. It is essential that the anesthetist know the conditions under which he or she is practicing, i.e., who is ultimately responsible, what kind of employment relationship exists, and, of great importance, what the type and adequacy of insurance coverage. These are concerns that need to be determined before and in the event of a lawsuit.

The legal climate changes as more verdicts and decisions are made and incorporated into the law. To keep abreast of these, the nurse anesthetist can read and study cases as they are decided. Cases of prime interest are those that reflect the opinions of the courts in given factual situations. They are primarily decisions of federal and state appellate courts, since, as a general rule, decisions of trial courts are not reported.

There are several sources from which to obtain information on legal cases that are of interest to anesthesia personnel. Looseleaf services such the *Professional Liability Newsletter,* published in Berkeley California, and the *Regan Report on Nursing Law,* published in Rhode Island are examples of sources of cases. These publications will often report on cases that were settled out of court, which would not be considered as precedent setting.

To aid the reader in understanding the legal lessons to be learned from the cases presented in this chapter, an analysis has been included at the end of most of the cases.

NEGLIGENCE—GALL BLADDER SURGERY

The patient, a 49-year-old female registered nurse, was having gall bladder surgery. About 2 hours into the operation, the surgeon advised the anesthesiologist that he could not feel a pulse. Emergency procedures were begun and the patient's heart responded almost immediately and then resumed its normal beat. From the operative notes, it appeared that her heart was at arrest for 5 minutes. The patient suffered permanent brain damage which left her partially blind, spastic, and unable to care for herself.

A negligence suit was filed against the anesthesiologist for failing to note that her heart was beating weakly and failing to take remedial measures before the cardiac arrest occurred.

Before the suit was filed, the anesthesiologist was notified by the patient's attorney that he wanted to examine the records of the operation. The anesthesiologist then began adding to the chart until he was advised by a clerk in the record room that his actions were improper.

The trial court judge instructed the jury that changes made on the chart were not material in determining the cause of the cardiac arrest. A verdict for the anesthesiologist was rendered by the jury. On appeal, the verdict for the anesthesiologist was reversed because the instructions regarding changes on the chart were in error. A new trial was ordered.

Seaton v. Rosenberg, 573 S.W. 2d 333 Ky. Sup. Ct. (1978)

Analysis. The lesson to be learned from this case is simple: it is legally unjustifiable to change notations on a patient's chart after the fact.

NEGLIGENCE—DENTAL ANESTHESIA

The patient underwent extraction of 23 teeth at the dentist's office in 1971. She filled out a brief form giving her medical history and signed a consent form on which she agreed to the operation and acknowledged that the nature and seriousness of the procedure had been explained to her. The dentist, who administered the anesthesia did not explain the possible risks of general anesthesia. The anesthesia given consisted of Demerol® [meperidine] 25 mg, atropine, 12 mg, and Brevital® [methohexital] 1 percent 15 cc. Oxygen 25 percent, nitrous oxide 75 percent, and Penthrane® [methoxyflurane] were then given.

During the recovery phase after the surgery, one of the dental assistants noticed that the patient was cyanotic and in cardiorespiratory arrest. The dentist attempted to revive her with drugs and chest massage. She was transferred to a hospital where she died 3 days later. The precise cause of her death was unknown as her parents refused to consent to an autopsy.

In a complaint in trespass filed by the patient's father, the trial court entered a verdict for the dentist. The plaintiff appealed and the higher court held that the trial court erred in refusing to instruct the jury on the question of informed consent. It appeared from the dentist's testimony that he did not discuss the risks of general anesthesia with the patient before she signed the consent form.

Sauro v. Shea, 390 2d Pa. Superior Ct. (1978)

Analysis. While the key issue as reported in the law book on this case is the lack of informed consent, the advisability of a dentist administering his own anesthesia and the competency of the personnel responsible for the patient's recovery is questionable. Perhaps this unfortunate accident would not have happened if there had been an anesthetist or anesthesiologist present.

NEGLIGENCE—SPINAL ANESTHETIC

On January 6, 1959, the plaintiff, a 67-year-old man, was admitted to the hospital for a hernia repair. The surgeon commented that the patient was in the best physical shape that he had ever seen him. A spinal anesthetic was administered by the surgeon. In administering the anesthetic, the surgeon instructed the patient to be perfectly still. Afterwards the plaintiff described the injection as follows: "When he put the needle in me, it was just like a strong electric current went through me, it just straightened me out, and I couldn't have prevented it no way. If there had been four people holding me I couldn't . . . it was just like lighting from the top of my head to the bottom of my toes."

Although the patient had received two spinals in the past, he said he never experienced anything like that before. A second injection of anesthetic was made without sensory experience to the plaintiff-patient. After the operation, and at the time of the trial, the patient had no sensory feeling from his naval to his knees and was unable to urinate without the use of tranquilizers and no longer experience a libidinal urge.

At the trial, medical expert witnesses, including a surgeon, urologist, neurologist, and an anesthesiologist, testified that the plaintiff's condition was beyond medical treatment. They also testified that the results were unusual, i.e. one would not expect a sensory loss from a spinal anesthetic.

The Superior Court of Benton County dismissed the medical malpractice action brought by the plaintiff. The dismissal was reversed and remanded for a new trial by the Court of Appeals.

The higher court ruled that there was sufficient circumstantial evidence for the jury to infer negligence under the doctrine of *res ipsa loquitur*. They said: "It is difficult to justifiably disregard application of the doctrine when a patient submits himself to the care and custody of medical personnel, is rendered unconscious, and receives some injury from instrumentalities used in his treatment. Without the aid of this doctrine, a patient who receives permanent injuries of a serious character, apparently the result of someone's negligence, would be unable to recover unless the doctors and nurses in attendance voluntarily chose to disclose the facts establishing liability."

Younger v. Webster, 510 P 2d 1182 90 ALR 3d 767 Wa. (1975)

Analysis. The court in this case recognized the vulnerability of patients receiving an anesthetic, who, having been rendered unconscious, are unable to testify as to the cause of the injury. By permitting a *re ipsa loquitur* holding, the fact that an injury occurred was sufficient in itself to infer negligence on the part of the medical personnel.

NEGLIGENCE—ANESTHESIA FOR EYE SURGERY

The plaintiff, a married, 48-year-old father of two children, was admitted to Kaiser Hospital for surgery to correct an obstruction of the tear sac on the right side of his eye. According to the hospital chart and the testimony of several nurses, nothing unusual occurred during the operation or the recovery period. When the patient was released from the hospital, he experienced spacial disorientation. He could no longer remember the location of things in the interior of his house. He had difficulty driving, a reduced field of vision, and a loss of memory.

The plaintiff was examined by several neurologists who determined that he had suffered permanent brain damage. He was fired from his job as a school teacher 1 year after the surgery because his memory was no longer sufficient. At the time of trial, his wage loss exceeded $45,000 and the jury was entitled to find that he had become virtually unemployable.

The expert witnesses for the plaintiff testified that the dose of narcotics given by the nurse anesthetist was "greatly excessive." They also testified that the medication given to counteract the anesthetic and to insure respiration was "insufficient in amount," and was not in accordance with "good medical practice." In addition, the expert witnesses testified that there "most probably was a period of respiratory depression after conclusion of the anesthetic in the recovery room." At that time, the "standing policy" of the defendant was to "count and observe" respiration of a patient in the recovery room and to administer oxygen, if needed, but *not* to chart such information unless something unusual was observed.

The Circuit Court rendered judgment on a jury verdict for the patient in the amount of $750,000 and the defendants appealed. The Oregon Supreme Court held that (1) evidence on the question of whether the hospital failed to reasonably monitor changes in the patient's respiration following surgery was sufficient for the jury, and that (2) the trial court did not err in excluding from the jury members of the group health plan of the clinic and hospital.

Wagner v. Kaiser Foundation Hospital, 589 P 2d 1106 Oregon (1979)

Analysis. While it is unfortunate that there are not more facts about the actual sequence of events during the anesthetic and postoperative care, it is clear that the lack of charting of respiration in the recovery room, made the case more difficult to defend.

NEGLIGENCE—LUMBAR LAMINECTOMY

"The patient, a 48-year-old laborer, experienced profound hypoxic brain damage incident to anesthesia for a lumbar laminectomy. On August 4, 1970, the patient had surgery under halothane and oxygen anesthesia; the concentration of halothane was reported to be 2 percent and total dose of 3 mg of curare was also given. The anesthesiologist controlled ventilation with a bag.

"Upon completion of the disc removal, and just as the patient was taken out of the jackknife position, his blood pressure dropped from 120 mm Hg systolic to 60. Vasoxy® [Methoxamine hydrochloride] was quickly administered and the systolic blood pressure more than doubled. At about this time, the assistant surgeon commented that the blood looked a little dark, and the anesthesiologist noted that the patient's nail beds were dusky.

"Because the pressure drop was brief and there was no arrhythmia or serious bradycardia, the doctors were not concerned. The patient was transported to the recovery room at 12:40 P.M. His respiration was spontaneous and adequate in depth. The recovery room nurse was not informed about the incident of cyanosis in the operating room.

"At 3:15 P.M., the nurse telephoned the anesthesiologist to inform him that the patient was still unconscious, that his heart rate was 140, and his arms and legs were rigid. A neurosurgeon was called at 3:30 P.M. when the patient developed opisthotonos. Appropriate treatment was given, but there was irreversible brain damage. The patient is currently in a rest home, bed-ridden, and profoundly obtunded.

"At the malpractice trial, the expert for the patient-plaintiff stressed the significance of cyanosis at the time of the hypotensive episode. Coupled with proof that the patient's brain damage was diffuse, and therefore most likely hypoxic in origin, his attorney was able to present a convincing argument that the hypoxia must have been due to inadequate ventilation during surgery. There was also testimony form the plaintiff's expert witness that

Legal Cases

the total dose of curare was too high (the patient weighed 160 pounds). He was particularly critical of the failure to constantly monitor respiration with a stethoscope. The anesthetic record was sparse, without any notaton of respiratory rate, although the anesthesiologist testified he checked respiration four or five times during the surgery.

"The hospital's liability was based on the recovery room nurse's failure to call a physician earlier when she recognized that the patient was not awakening and was becoming rigid. The hospital settled out of court for $75,000 shortly before the trial began. The trial took 16 days and the jury was out 1½ days. They awarded the plaintiff $433,000 in damages."

Monterey County Superior Court No. 70429, from Rubsamen D: Professional Liability Newsletter, 1X, No. 9, March, 1978 Reprinted with permission.

Analysis. A key element in this case was inadequate continuous monitoring of heart and ventilation, as well as poor charting on the anesthesia record which made the case difficult to defend.

CARDIAC ARREST—EYE SURGERY

"On December 7, 1974, the patient, a 26-year-old man, entered a California hospital shortly after he was accidentally shot in the eye with a pellet gun. He was immediately taken to surgery for repair of a corneal laceration. During the course of the anesthesia there was a cardiac arrest. Although the patient was resuscitated, he suffered severe brain damage and died 7 days later.

"At the malpractice trial the cause of the cardiac arrest was never determined. The defense postulated a particularly strong vagal reflex from manipulation of the eye. The plaintiff claimed there was a period of oxygen deprivation prior to the arrest, possibly from intubation of the right main stem bronchus, but no atelectasis was identified in the left lung.

"There was considerable testimony about the erratic behavior of the anesthesiologist during the 2 months prior to the malpractice incident. It was contended that he had been found asleep on the floor on one occasion and had fallen asleep in the cafeteria at another time, and that on more than one additional occasion he had appeared to be sedated. All of this testimony was relevant to the malpractice incident, because a physician called to the OR when the cardiac arrest occurred, testified that the defendant was not responding to the emergency, but seemed "trance like" and inert. There was contradictory evidence from the OR nurses and the surgeon who said the defendant's performance was normal.

"The anesthesiologist did not attend the trial as he died in a fire in his apartment a week after the anesthesia accident. At the time of his death, multiple needle marks were found on his arm. The senior anesthesiologist who had hired him was also named in the suit, based on empoyer-employee liability. The senior man had recruited his associate and there was evidence of an employment contract with a compensation arrangement based on gross income. There was further contention that the senior anesthesiologist should have noted his colleague's drug-related problems and taken appropriate action.

"The jury was out 9 hours following a 5-week trial. The senior anesthesiologist, the dead anesthesiologist's estate, and the hospital were found liable. Damages of $834,790 were awarded to the parents and the wife of the patient."

Alameda County Superior Court No. 460898-3, from Rubsamen D: Professional Liability Newsletter, 1X, No. 9, March 1978. Reprinted with permission.

Analysis. This case illustrates two points of negligence: that of the anesthesiologist who actually administered the anesthesia and that of the senior anesthesiologist and the hospital for failing to take corrective action as soon as any erratic behavior was noticed. The finding of liability against both the anesthesiologist and the hospital is evidence that in the health care field, an employer has a *legal* responsibility to demand that employees maintain high standards of professional conduct.

NEGLIGENCE—OB REGIONAL ANESTHESIA

"The patient, a 17-year-old mother, was admitted to the hospital in June, 1976 for delivery. A nurse, who had been working at the hospital for one week, was on duty in the obstetrical department. She was foreign born and could speak only a little English.

"A few minutes after admission, the nurse telephoned the family physician to report that the cervix was dilated to 9 cm and that the head was at zero station. The doctor arrived at 4:30 A.M. and noted the head was at a plus 2 station and there was crowning with contractions. Five minutes later he performed a saddle block. Immediately after the block was administered, the patient was placed on the delivery table. While the doctor was placing sterile drapes, approximately 4 minutes after the block, the nurse testified the she observed the patient was attempting to talk but couldn't, and a minute later she told the doctor that the patient could not breathe, but he did not respond appropriately.

"The nurse called her supervisor and told her the patient could not breathe. A code blue was called and the supervisor began mouth to mouth resuscitation. The apnea was followed by a cardiac arrest. It was unclear from the record just how soon the code blue team arrived, and there was a problem in obtaining adequate equipment. An endotracheal tube was not inserted until 5:04 A.M. Delivery was at 6:06 with low forceps. The baby was cyanotic and responded poorly. The mother remained comatose and died 5 days later. The child, at age 2½, cannot sit, crawl, or hold up her head.

"The malpractice suit was settled out of court with the following damages awarded: A $500,000 lump sum payment, plus $2,500 per month to the injured child for life with a guaranteed 10-year minimum, regardless of her survival.

"If the case had gone to trial, the defense would have postulated that the complication was due to pulmonary embolism. The plaintiff's attorney felt that it could be proved that the patient did not move, beginning with the time she was unable to speak, which would support the conclusion that she was paralyzed from a complete spinal anesthetic."

Los Angeles Superior Court No. SOC 45750, from Rubsamen D: Professional Liability Newsletter, X, No. 7, February 1979. Reprinted with permission.

Analysis. This case shows clearly that only professionals trained in anesthesia should be administering the techniques and monitoring the patients. This was a *needless* death!

NEGLIGENCE—ENT SURGERY

"On May 5, 1975, a 4-year-old child underwent bilateral myringotomy and an adnoidectomy because of repeated ear infections and hypertrophied adnoids. A first year resident performed the surgery and the anesthetic was administered by a nurse anesthetist. The myringotomies were performed first. The resident recovered only a few strips of tissue in the course of the adnoidectomy. The chief of ENT was not present for the myringotomies, and there was conflicting testimony as to whether he arrived before or just after the adnoidectomy was accomplished. At any rate, he saw the strips of tissue on a gauze sponge, remarked that there didn't seem to be "enough tissue here" and, as he testified later, looked for more tissue in the pharynx, found none, and palpated the surgical area and noted that it was clean. The patient was then extubated and placed on a guerney.

"As the child took his first breath, he choked and became cyanotic. A code blue was called and a scrub nurse ran from the room to obtain a bronchoscope. She returned and handed the instrument to the chief of ENT. He was about to insert it when the chief of anesthesiology came into the room in response to the code blue. It was the anesthesiologist's impression that a bronchospasm accounted for the problem, so he advised against inserting a bronchoscope as this could aggravate the spasm. The instrument was put aside and the brochoscopy was not reconsidered.

"The endotracheal tube was reinserted and the patient was given oxygen. Efforts to relieve the complication were continuous, including the administration of epinephrine twice. A chest x-ray indicated a bilateral pneumothorax which was treated with chest tubes. A pericardial tamponade was suspected, but an attempt at aspiration produced no blood. The child died. An autopsy revealed two lumps of adenoidal tissue [in the trachea], each approximately 2½ by ¾ of an inch in area and 1 inch thick, weighing a total of 2.2 grams.

"At trial, the plaintiff's attorney had no problem with the standard of care issue. The failure to perform a bronchoscopy, once large doses of epinephrine did not alleviate the presumed bronchospasm, was regarded by the jury as an especially critical oversight. In his testimony, the chief of ENT conceded his judgment error in this regard.

"The pathologist testified that relief of the obstruction, even a matter of minutes before death, probably would have resulted in complete recovery, since he felt there was no microscopic evidence of irreversible brain damage.

"Several months before the trial, the defense offered $140,000 in settlement, but the parents refused. On the day of the trial, the parents decided to accept the offer, but the defense would not tender their offer a second time. The jury awarded a verdict of $300,000 for the death of the child."

Alameda County Superior Court No. 478735, reported in Rubsamen D: Professional Liability Newsletter, XII, No. 3, December 1980. Reprinted with permission.

NEGLIGENCE—GYNECOLOGIC SURGERY

"The decedent, a 25-year-old mother of three children entered the hospital for a tubal ligation and incidental appendectomy on January 29, 1975. She was 5 feet, 3 inches tall and weighed 200 pounds. The preoperative medication was Demerol® [meperidine] 100 mg, Vistaril® [hydroxyzine pamoate] 100 mg, and Scopolamine 0.4 mg. Anesthesia consisted of Pentothal® [thiopental], nitrous oxide, and Anectine® [succinylcholine chloride]. There was no endotracheal intubation noted on the anesthetic records, although the doctor recalled that this was done. He also said that

Legal Cases

the patient's breathing was spontaneous throughout the procedure with an "occasional" assistance of respiration by bag breathing. Monitoring was by ECG.

"Surgery began at 7:30 A.M., 15 minutes after anesthesia induction. The surgeon immediately commented that the blood seemed dark and the anesthesiologist administered 100 percent oxygen for a brief period until the blood became a normal color once more. At 8:35 A.M., the patient experienced a severe bradycardia for 3 minutes and this was followed by asystole. Cardiopulmonary resuscitation was immediately initiated and the heart's rhythm was restored after 32 minutes. However the patient did not recover consciousness and died at 6:15 P.M. the next day.

"At trial, the plaintiff's expert witness noted the increased anesthetic risk created by the patient's size and criticized the failure to intubate her or employ ventilatory assistance, especially since she had received Anectine®. It was contended that these omissions resulted in progressive hypoxia which led to the cardiac arrest. Once the arrest occurred, it was asserted that the anesthesiologist was unskilled in dealing with it.

The defense case was based on a theory that the cardiac arrest had nothing to do with hypoxia. There was evidence that the patient had taken a variety of reducing medications since 1968. For 30 days before surgery she had been on dextroamphetamine 15 mg and Compazine® [prochlorperazine] 7.5 mg. She was also taking thyroid and Diuril® [chlorothiazide] daily and Seconal® [secobarbital] at bedtime. It was the surgeon who had given the patient her prescription for these drugs, but neither he nor the patient had informed the anesthesiologist about this medication.

"The anesthesia record did not reflect progressive hypoxia, and the defense expert witnesses said the abrupt onset of the cardiac arrest preceded by severe bradycardia was consistent with a synergistic effect between the anesthetic drugs and the medications she was taking. The risk of liability for the surgeon and assistant surgeon mainly concerned their failure to take more aggressive and appropriate action in managing the cardiac arrest.

"The hospital was also named as a defendant. It was the plaintiff's theory that the nurses were not well trained in CPR. Also, it was contended that since the anesthesiologist received his instruction entirely by preceptorship, he was poorly qualified and should have been excluded from the hospital staff. However, the judge granted the hospital's motion for a nonsuit after the plaintiff's case. . . .

"The surgeon and assistant surgeon made an out of court settlement for $175,000 just before the trial began. The jury awarded a $1,159,000 verdict against the *uninsured* anesthesiologist."

Los Angeles County Superior Court, No. NOC–1896, from Rubsamen D: Professional Liability Newsletter, XII, No. 3, December 1980. Reprinted with permission.

NEGLIGENCE—ORTHOPEDIC SURGERY

"The plaintiff-patient, who was 14 years old, was injured in a motorcycle accident December 31, 1975. He was taken to a nearby community hospital, arriving there at 6:10 P.M. Although he had been initially unconscious for about 10 minutes, the examining physician found him to be alert. He exhibited mutiple soft tissue injuries and his right tibia as well as his right ulna and radus were broken. A supine chest film revealed consolidation at both lung bases. It was believed that this reflected contusions of his lungs.

"The patient was transferred to a university hospital at 10:25 P.M. and was immediately examined by a second year neurosurgical resident. The resident testified later in a deposition that the x-ray evidence of lung contusions led him to the conclusion that the patient had a substantial risk of spontaneous pneumothorax, on one or both sides, over the next 8 hours. At midnight, a first year resident took over from the neurosurgical resident, and at 3:15 A.M. the patient was taken to surgery to have his fractures reduced.

"Anesthetic induction was carried out by the chief of anesthesiology and then he turned the case over to a student nurse anesthetist who was in her second year of training. The chief then left the OR. At the conclusion of the surgery, 5:30 A.M., the student anesthetist asked her chief to check the patient again, which he did. He ventilated him, noted he appeared stable and told the anesthetist to leave the tube in for awhile. Because there was no recovery room space available, the patient was taken directly to the orthopedic floor, accompanied by the nurse anesthetist and the orthopedic resident. They arrived on the ward at 5:40 P.M.

"The ward nurse noticed that the patient's respirations were "loud, noisy, and wet." The nurse anesthetist stayed with the patient. About 5:15 A.M. the patient began to "buck" against the endotracheal tube and, just as it was removed, he experienced a cardiac arrest. Although resuscitation was effective, the patient remained in a coma for 6 weeks. His recovery was complicated by a subscapsular splenic hematoma, which required surgery on the afternoon of January 1, 1976. The following day the Ohio Ventilator, to which the patient was attached, failed. Bag breathing was necessary for 20 minutes. He had some pupillary reflexes before this, but none afterward.

"The patient's subsequent recovery had been good with regard to motor deficit and he only has a foot drop on the left. His intellectual loss, however, is substantial. His I.Q., previously 93, is now 65 and his short-term memory is particularly bad. He lives at home with his mother.

"An out of court settlement was agreed upon. A lump sum of $350,000 was paid and the attorney's fee will come out of that. The patient will receive $1,500 a month for life. At age 25, he will receive a payment of

$25,000 and at 35, a payment of $35,000. Thereafter these payments will be increased by $10,000 jumps every 5 years.

San Bernardino Superior Court, No. 174929, from Rubsamen D: Professional Liability Newsletter, XIII, No. 3, January, 1982. Reprinted with permission.

Analysis. The recovery of the anesthetized patient must be of primary concern to the profession. The anesthetist has a legal duty to remain with the patient until her care is no longer required. The care of the patient should then be turned over only to qualified personnel.

NEGLIGENCE—PNEUMOENCEPHALOGRAM

"A 29-year-old telephone repair man suffered brain damage incident to a cardiac arrest which occurred in the course of a pneumoencephalogram. The patient had a skull x-ray in 1974, and an incidental finding was an enlarged sella turcica. A year later, a repeat skull film again demonstrated the abnormality. Since he was symptom free, it was decided to observe him. Over the next 3 years there developed progressive changes of acromegaly. When the patient entered the hospital, May 15, 1978, his mandible was greatly enlarged, and he had severe macroglossia; the tongue was almost twice the normal size. This caused a partial airway obstruction when he slept in certain positions.

"An intrasellar mass was identified and a pneumoencephalogram was scheduled to define the precise boundries of the lesion. A nurse anesthetist and a radiologist were present for the procedure. The patient received Valium® [diazepam] and Compazine® [prochlorperazine] at noon followed by droperidol at 1:00 P.M. Nisentil® [alphaprodine] was selected as the narcotic of choice. The nurse diluted 40 mg of Nisentil® in 10 cc of solution and administered about half of it intravenously in divided doses between 1:05 and 1:30 P.M. The patient was in a sitting position with his head flexed.

"At 2:00 P.M. the radiologist made the initial spinal tap. Air was injected for the first time at 2:15 P.M. In his deposition, the nurse anesthetist said that just before this the patient's chest movement suggested "a degree of hypoventilation." This lasted about 2 minutes. However, he did not call this to the attention of the radiologist, and did not manipulate the patient's jaw in order to improve the airway.

"The radiologist stated in depostion that at about 2:15 P.M., he felt the patient's nail beds were dusky. He concluded that there was hypoxia and asked the anesthetist if the patient was ventilating properly. He was told "Yes," and he did not pursue the question further.

"The anesthetist had assisted ventilation with a face mask and attached bag. No oropharyngeal airway was inserted. After a period of hypoventilation, he taped the mask to the patient's face, and, since he felt there was no further problem with breathing, he discontinued ventilatory assistance. Several x-rays were taken between 2:15 and 2:45 P.M., at which time the patient became pale but not cyanotic.

"With the patient still in a sitting position, the anesthetist began assisting respiration by squeezing the bag attached to the face mask. Within a few minutes he noted a marked resistance to pressure on the bag. An anesthesiologist was called and he arrived 3 or 4 minutes later, just as the patient became profoundly cyanotic and experienced a cardiac arrest.

"During the entire procedure the patient was attached to an ECG monitor, and the anesthetist stated that he checked his pulse, blood pressure, and respirations every couple of minutes. He said there was no alteration in vital signs at any time before the caridac arrest, although there were premature ventricular contractions of the ECG a about 2:45 P.M.

"Resuscitation was prompt, but the patient manifested severe, acute brain damage. He was comatose for about 3 weeks during which time he had frequent myoclonic seizures. He then slowly recovered and regained his full intellectual capacity. However, he has muscle dysarthia, can only walk with assistance, and has some spacity of both arms. He spends most of his time in a wheelchair. He is not employable.

"An out of court settlement was made in this case. Had the case been tried, the plaintiff's expert witnesses would have developed two major negligence issues. First, because of the patient's macroglossia, the anesthetist should have anticipated an airway problem following the preliminary sedation and the adminstration of Nisentil®. Second, the plaintiff's expert witness would have raised a question about adequate monitoring, contending the cardiac arrest probably was not suddenly manifested without a preceding change in vital signs. The anesthetist would have been charged with unreasonable delay in acting to relieve the airway obstruction which presumably was due to the patient's large tongue.

"The settlement was arranged in the following manner: The patient was paid $500,000 in a lump sum, plus $45,000 to cover his lost income and expenses. He will then receive $15,000 for lost wages between July 1, 1980 and July 1, 1981. At this later date his annuities will begin. This will be $30,000 per year, compounded at 3 percent annually. The payments are tax free. There is aguarantee of 20 years, regardless of whether the patient lives that long. The attorney's fees, paid in addition to the settlement, were $300,000."

Santa Clara County Superior Court, No. 426391, from Rubsamen D: Professional liability Newsletter, XI, No. 10, June 1980. Reprinted with permission.

Legal Cases 119

DENTAL ANESTHESIA

"The patient, a 56-year-old man died 10 days after dental extraction performed under general anesthesia. He received I.V. sodium pentothal administered by a nurse anesthetist. Following the procedure, gauze squares were placed on the bleeding gums. After the packs were in place, the patient recovered consciousness enough to he helped to a recovery area where he was seated in a chair.

"The recovery area was staffed by a young woman without any formal nursing training. After an uncertain period, the patient was found slumped over in the chair in respiratory arrest. The nurse anesthetist attempted to resuscitate the patient while leaving him upright in the chair. She testified in deposition, that she inserted an endotracheal tube.

"An ambulance was called; when the crew arrived, they placed the patient on the floor and administered CPR after removing the gauze packing from his mouth. Although resuscitation was successful, the patient was completely unresponsive with fixed, dilated pupils. The nurse said one of the ambulance crew removed the endotracheal tube.

"The patient was then taken to a nearby hospital, where an endotracheal tube was again inserted and he was placed on a ventilator. A few days later a tracheostomy was performed. His arterial blood gases were essentially normal, along with normal chest x-rays. However, he failed to regain consciousness and died on the tenth hospital day.

"At autopsy, a gauze square was found in the trachea. There was no radio-opaque line in the gauze, so it did not show up in the chest films.

"A malpractice action was filed by the widow and adult children of the patient. It was the plaintiff's theory that the patient aspirated the gauze shortly after he was placed in the recovery area in the dentist's office. Presumably he was so obtunded by the anesthetic that he was unable to cough it up. It was postulated this respiratory obstruction accounted for the brain damage before the anesthetist inserted an endotracheal tube.

"The case was settled out of court for $400,000, with the insurance carriers for the dentist and anesthetist contributing $200,000."

Los Angeles County Superior Court, No. SEC–21763 (California) from Professional Liability Newsletter, November 1979. Reprinted with permission.

Analysis. A good lesson can be learned from this case: it is important to assure that all personnel present in anesthesia and postanesthesia areas are well trained and qualified.

Glossary of Legal Terms

ad damnum. The amount of damages demanded.

adversary proceeding. A proceeding involving a real controversy contested by two opposing parties.

agency. Relation in which one person acts on behalf of another with the authority of the latter.

agent. One who by mutual consent acts for the benefit of another.

aggrieved party. One who has been injured or suffered a loss.

amicus curiae. Friend of the court, one who gives information to the court on some matter of law that is in doubt.

answer. The principle pleading on the part of the defendant in response to plaintiff's complaint.

antitrust laws. Statutes such as the Sherman Antitrust Act, directed against unlawful restraints of trade and monopolies.

appellant. The party who appeals a decision, or who brings the proceeding to a reviewing court.

appellate court. A court having jurisdiction to review the law as applied to a prior determination of the same case.

appellee. The party who argues, on appeal, against the setting aside of the judgement.

assault. An attempt, with unlawful force, to inflict bodily injury upon another, accompanied by the apparent present ability to give effect to the attempt if not prevented.

assignment. Act whereby one transfers one's interest in a right or property to another.

attorney general. The chief law officer of the federal government or of each state government.

bargaining unit. A group of employees recognized by the employer, or certified by an administrative agency, as appropriate for the purpose of representation by a union through collective bargaining. All employees in the appropriately designated unit are covered by subsequent collective bargaining agreements negotiated.

battery. The unlawful touching of another without their consent.

beneficiary. One receiving or designated to receive benefit or advantage.

breach of contract. A failure to perform for which legal excuse is lacking.

breach of duty. Failure to perform a duty owed to another.

brief. A written argument concentrating upon legal points and authorities, used by a lawyer to convey to the court the essential facts of the case.

cause of action. A claim in law and fact sufficient to demand judicial attention.

certiorari. A means of gaining appelllate review.

circumstantial evidence. Indirect evidence, secondary facts by which a principal fact may be rationally inferred.

civil law. That branch of law that pertains to suits outside of criminal.

civil rights. Rights given, defined, and circumscribed by positive laws enacted by civilized communities.

class action. A lawsuit brought by representative members of a large group of persons on behalf of all members of the group.

common law. The system of jurisprudence, which originated in England and was later applied in the United States, which is based on judicial *precedent* rather than legislative enactment.

comparative negligence. The proportional sharing between plaintiff and defendant of compensation of injuries based on the relative negligence of the two.

consideration (contract law). One element of a contract that is generally required to make a promise binding and to make the agreement of the parties enforceable as a contract.

consortium. The conjugal fellowship of husband and wife and the right of each to the company, cooperation, and aid of the other in every conjugal relation.

contributory negligence. Conduct on the part of the *plaintiff* which falls below the standard to which he should conform and which is a legally contributing cause with the negligence of the defendant in bringing about the plaintiff's harm.

defendant. In civil proceedings, the party being sued.

defense. A denial, answer, or plea opposing truth or validity of plaintiff's case

demurrer. Formal allegation that the facts, as stated in the pleadings, are not legally sufficient for the case to proceed any further.

deposition. A method of pretrial discovery that consists of a statement of a witness, under oath, taken in question and answer form.

directed verdict. That verdict returned by the jury at the direction of the trial judge, by whose instruction the jury is bound.

discovery. Pretrial procedure by which the parties gain vital information concerning the case.

dismissal. Equivalent of a cancellation.

due care. A concept used in tort law to indicate the standard of care or the legal duty one owes to others.

evidence. All the means by which alleged matter of fact is established or disproved.

finding. Decision of the court on issues of facts.

fraud. Intentional deception resulting in injury to another.

gross negligence. Failure to use even slight care (see negligence).

hearsay rule. Evidence of a statement which is made other than by a witness while testifying at the hearing, offered to prove the truth of the matter stated.

impute. To assign to a person or other entity, such as an employer, the legal responsibility for the act of another.

informed consent. Consent given only after full notice is given, such as nature and risk of a procedure.

injunction. A judicial remedy for the purpose of requiring a party to refrain from doing a particular act or activity.

joint liability. Such shared liability as results in the right of any one party sued to insist that others be sued jointly with him.

joint tort-feasors. Two or more persons who owe to another the same duty and whose negligence results in injury to such other person, thus rendering the tort-feasors both jointly and individually liable for the injury.

judge-made law. Law made in common law by precedent rather than statute.

jurisdiction. The power to hear and determine a case.

liability. An obligation to do or refrain from doing something.

litigation. A judicial contest through which legal rights are determined and enforced.

mitigation of damages. A requirement that one injured by reason of another's tort or breach of agreement, exercise reasonable diligence and ordinary care to avoid aggravating the injury or increasing damages.

motion. An application to the court requesting an order or rule in favor of the applicant.

negligence. Failure to exercise that degree of care which a person of ordinary prudence would exercise under the same or similar circumstances.

nonsuit. A judgment rendered against a plaintiff who fails to proceed to trial or who is unable to prove his case.

offer. A promise, a commitment to do or refrain from doing some specific thing in the future.

opinion. The reason given for a court's judgment, finding, or conclusion, as opposed to the *decision*, which is the judgment itself.

pain and suffering. A type of damage that one may receive for physical or mental "pain and suffering" that resulted from a wrong done.

Glossary

plaintiff. The one who initially brings suit.

precedent. Previously decided case which is recognized as an authority for the disposition of future cases.

product liability. Tort law which dictates that a manufacturer is strictly liable for articles placed on the market.

question of law. Disputed legal contentions which are traditionally left for the judge to decide.

remedy. The means employed to enforce or redress an injury.

res ipsa loquitur. The thing speaks for itself: negligence may be inferred from the mere fact that the accident happened. Provisions apply.

respondeat superior. Let the superior reply. Liability of employer for the acts of employee.

reversal. The setting aside, annulling, vacating, or changing the decision of a lower court or other body.

scope of employment. The range of activities encompassed by one's employment.

settlement. The conclusive fixing or resolving of a matter.

stare decisis. To stand by what is decided (see precedent).

statute. An act of the legislature adopted pursuant to its constitutional authority.

statute of limitations. Any law that fixes the time within which parties must take judicial action to enforce rights or else be thereafter barred from enforcing them.

strict liability. Liability without a showing of fault.

summary judgment. Preverdict judgment rendered by the court in response to a motion by plaintiff or defendant, who claims that the absence of factual dispute on one or more issues eliminates the need to send those issues to the jury.

tort. A wrong, private or civil, resulting from a breach of legal duty.

unfair labor practice. Union or employer tactics classified as "unfair" under federal or state labor laws.

vicarious liability. The imputation of liability upon one person for the actions of another.

witness. One who gives evidence in a cause before a court and who attests or swears to facts or gives or bears testimony under oath.

wrongful death statute. Statutes that provide that an action can be maintained for any wrongful act, neglect, or default which causes death.

Appendixes

Appendix A
Statute of Limitations

State	Years	Comments
Alabama	2	
Alaska	2	
Arizona	3	
Arkansas	2	
California	3	In no event shall the time for commencement of legal actions exceed 3 years except upon proof of fraud, intentional concealment, or presence of foreign body.
Colorado	3	
Connecticut	1	
Delaware	2	
District of Columbia	3	
Florida	2	Extended 2 years for fraud, concealment, or intentional misrepresentation.
Georgia	2	
Hawaii	2	
Idaho	2	
Illinois	2	
Indiana	2	
Iowa	2	
Kansas	2	
Kentucky	1	
Louisiana	1	
Maine	2	
Maryland	5	
Massachusetts	3	
Michigan	2	
Minnesota	2	
Mississippi	2	
Missouri	2	
Montana	3	
Nebraska	2	
Nevada	4	
New Hampshire	2	
New Jersey	2	
New Mexico	3	
New York	2½	

Statute of Limitations

North Carolina	2	Cause of action for malpractice shall be deemed to accrue at the time of the occurrence of the defendant giving rise to the cause of actions
North Dakota	2	
Ohio	1	
Oklahoma	2	
Oregon	2	
Pennsylvania	2	
Rhode Island	2	
South Carolina	3	
South Dakota	2	
Tennessee	1	
Texas	2	
Utah	2	
Vermont	3	
Virginia	2	
Washington	3	
West Virginia	2	
Wisconsin	3	
Wyoming	2	

Appendix B
Basic Structure of the Union Contract: A Sample Outline

I. Preamble
   A. Purpose of the contract
   B. Cooperation between nurses' union and hospital
   C. Parties to the agreement

II. Recognition
   A. Types of union recognition
      1. Craft wide (by occupation)
      2. Industrial
   B. Reference to specific bargaining unit
      1. Inclusions in the bargaining unit
      2. Exclusions in the bargaining unit
   C. Union recognition following hospital expansion, consolidation, or successor arrangements

III. Union Security Arrangements
   A. Types of arrangements
      1. Open shop
      2. Union shop
      3. Maintenance of membership
      4. Agency fee (fair share)
      5. Other combinations
   B. Payroll deduction—check-off of union dues
   C. Definition of union member in "good standing"
   D. Work of the nurses' bargaining unit work
      1. Definition of work
      2. Job description
      3. Subcontracting of bargaining unit work
         a. Use of students and volunteers
         b. Use of supervisors
         c. Use of medical pool personnel

IV. Hospital Hiring Procedures
   A. Staff nurses employed
      1. Numbers to be employed
      2. Nurse-patient ratios
         a. Patient Classifications
         b. Qualifications of needed personnel
      3. Procedure for employment of nurses
      4. Orientation of newly employed nurses
         a. To hospital
         b. To union

Outline of Sample Union Contract

  B. Definition of employee status
   1. Full-time employee
   2. Part-time employee
   3. Temporary employee
   4. Probationary employee
      a. Length of probation
      b. Rights of probationary employee

V. Hours of Work
   A. Definition of work day and work week
   B. Definition of shifts
   C. Guaranteed hours of work for bargaining unit
   D. Schedule of work
      1. Time frame for posting of work schedules
      2. Notification procedures for changes in posted work schedule
      3. Shift selection by seniority

VI. Rates of Pay
   A. Determination of pay rates
      1. Negotiated salary step system
         a. Length of service only
         b. Merit increase only (based on evaluations)
            1. Process to determine merit increase
            2. Who determines process
         c. Length of service if work is satisfactory
            1. Determined by whom
            2. Process for service accrual
         d. Time schedule for step increases
      2. Bargaining plus merit system
      3. Escalator clause based on cost of living
      4. Education advancement
   B. Pay schedules
      1. Hourly or weekly rate
      2. Annual salary schedule
   C. Shift differential
   D. Overtime provisions
      1. Definition of overtime
         a. Over 8 hours in 1 day
         b. Over 40 hours in 1 week
         c. Saturday and holidays
         d. Before or after scheduled and posted shift assignments
         e. Method for paying calculated overtime

2. Record keeping of overtime
     a. Calculation of overtime
     b. No layoff to offset individual accrual of overtime
     c. Records open to union
  3. Definition of double time
     a. Over 16 hours in 1 day
     b. Sundays
     c. Over 8 hours on Saturday
     d. Emergency transport of patients
     e. Methods for paying calculated double time
  4. Mandatory or voluntary overtime
  5. Assignment of overtime
     a. On basis of best qualified
     b. On basis of seniority only
     c. On request basis only
     d. Rotation plan
     e. On basis of seniority or specific patient unit
     f. Other combination
  6. Pay limit to only one basis of calculating overtime (pyramiding)
E. Out of classification pay (charge nurse or temporary supervisory placement)
  1. Minimum hours to be paid
  2. Length of temporary assignment
F. Call-in pay
  1. Scheduling of call duty
     a. On basis of seniority on patient area
     b. Preference only
     c. Rotation plan
  2. Notice for assignment of call-duty
  3. Minimum hours to be paid
  4. Number of hours guaranteed for call-in-time
  5. Relationship of call-in duty and overtime provisions
G. Pay periods
  1. Weekly
  2. Biweekly
  3. Monthly
H. Severance pay
  1. Inclusions
     a. Time worked
     b. Accrued but unused vacation
     c. Accrued but unused sick leave
  2. In event of no notice from hospital
     a. Pay for number of posted hours scheduled to work

b. Flat sum
c. Percentage of annual earnings
d. Based on years of service
e. Other combinations

VII. Evaluations
  A. Time frame for evaluations
    1. Advance notice requirement
    2. Annual on date of employment
  B. Content of evaluation
    1. Determined by whom
    2. Approved by whom
  C. Process for evaluation
    1. Evaluated by immediate supervisor or someone of similar occupational background
    2. Evaluation subject to grievance procedure
    3. Staff nurse access to personnel file

VII. Holidays
  A. Specific list and dates of holidays
  B. Eligibility requirements for holiday pay
    1. Length of service
    2. Dates of accrual
    3. Prorate for part-time employees
  C. Preferential requests for holiday
    1. Request only
    2. Seniority only
  D. Amount of holiday pay
    1. Rates of pay
      a. Straight time
      b. Straight time plus shift differential
      c. Overtime provisions
    2. Number of paid hours per holiday
    3. Holidays which fall on scheduled workday
      a. Overtime plus compensatory time off
      b. Time frame for use of compensatory time off
  E. Holiday falls during scheduled vacation
    1. Extra day off
    2. Extra pay

IX. Vacation
  A. Amount of vacation
    1. Determination of vacation
      a. According to years of service

        b. According to the number of days worked
    2. Vacation for part-time nurses
  B. Eligibility for use of yacation
    1. Length of service
    2. Number of hours worked in given time period
    3. Use of vacation time in conjunction with leave of absence
    4. Use of vacation time accrued during lay-off, accident, or illness, or strikes
  C. Accrual of vacation
  D. Calculation of vacation pay
    1. Hourly
    2. Straight time plus shift differential
    3. Percentage of annual earnings
    4. Other
  E. Use of vacation time
    1. Choice of vacation by seniority
      a. Hospital wide
      b. According to assigned patient unit
    2. Procedure for split vacation time
    3. Process for requesting vacation
    4. Process for scheduling vacation
  F. Reimbursement for accrued by unused vacation time
    1. Death of nurse
    2. Undisputed discharge
    3. Voluntary termination
    4. Extended lay-off or disability

X. Sick Leave
  A. Number of sick leave days
    1. Based on number of hours worked
    2. Based on number of 8-hour days worked
    3. Quarterly adjustment for full-time nurses
    4. Flat number annually
    5. Other combination
  B. Eligibility for use of sick leave
    1. From date of employment
    2. After probation period
  C. Accrual of sick leave
  D. Pay schedule for sick leave
    1. Straight time
    2. Straight time plus shift differential

XI. In-Service Education
  A. Scheduling and posting of in-service programs

Outline of Sample Union Contract

    B. Paid time for attendance
    C. Content of in-service education programs
       1. Determined by whom
       2. Approved by whom
       3. Presented by whom

XII. Seniority
    A. Method for determining seniority
       1. By job classification
       2. By department
       3. Hospital wide
       4. Other combination
    B. Calculation of seniority
       1. Date of hire at facility
       2. Date of actual employment
       3. Last date of return to work
       4. Date of hire in specific job classification
       5. Accumulation of seniority during lay-off, leaves of absence, job-related disability, strikes
       6. Other combination
    C. Seniority lists
       1. Preparation of lists
       2. Time period for preparation
       3. Dates for delivery of lists to union
       4. Posting of seniority lists
       5. Method for correcting seniority lists
    D. Termination of seniority
       1. Undisputed discharge from hospital
       2. Unauthorized leave of absence
       3. Lay-off in excess of specified period of time
       4. Failure to return to work within specified number of days after recall
       5. Failure to return after scheduled leave of absence
       6. Voluntary termination
       7. Other

XIII. Lay-Off and Recall
    A. Notification to union of impending lay-off
    B. Negotiation over impact of lay-off
    C. Lay-off by reverse seniority
       1. Hospital wide
       2. By patient unit
       3. By job classification

4. By job qualification
   a. Determined by whom
   b. Approved by whom
5. "Bumping" rights
   a. Notification of nurses involved
   b. Time limits
   c. Number of bumps
   d. Option for lay-off over bumping
   e. Job orientation for nurses in new jobs
D. Maintenance of seniority in lay-off
E. Recall notification to union and nurses involved
F. Process for recall
   1. Seniority only
   2. Qualification only
   3. By patient unit assigned
   4. Combination of above
   5. Secure nurses' rights to original job on recall
   6. Provision that all nurses laid off are rehired before new applicants sought
      a. Qualifications
      b. Consolidation of facilities or patient units
      c. Orientation to new job
      d. Other
G. Determine time frame of recall
H. Penalties for nurses who do not return when recalled
   1. Time limits
   2. Exceptions
   3. Other

XIV. Job Posting, Promotion, and Transfer
A. Posting of all job openings
   1. Content of posted job openings
      a. Job description
      b. Salary classification
      c. Qualifications
   2. Posting for "inside" applicants before hiring from outside
   3. Time frame for posting
   4. Site for job postings
B. Process for bidding on posted jobs
   1. Time frame
   2. Application for opening
      a. Verbal vs written
      b. Copies to union

Outline of Sample Union Contract

      3. Restrictions on eligibility
         a. Time between job changes
         b. Length of service
         c. Exclusions of temporary or probationary nurses
         d. Other
    C. Filling of posted positions
      1. Process
         a. Seniority only
         b. Qualification and ability
         c. Most senior nurse qualified
         d. Combination of above
      2. Final decision-maker on all nurse openings
      3. Time limit for nurse placement into open job
      4. Application of trial period
         a. Orientation to new job
         b. Length of trial period
         c. Evaluation of trial period
            1. By whom
            2. Time frame for evaluation
            3. Content of evaluation
    D. Temporary vacancies
      1. Definition
      2. Posting of all vacancies
         a. Job description
         b. Hours of work
         c. Rates of pay
         d. Qualification
      3. Time period vacancy may be considered temporary
      4. Job orientation before placement
      5. Advance written notification of temporary transfers

XV. Leaves of Absence
    A. Paid leaves
      1. Disability
      2. Personal days
      3. Union business and convention
      4. Jury duty
      5. Military reserve duty
      6. Continuing education days
      7. Bereavement
      8. Special education programs
      9. Other

B. Unpaid leaves
   1. Paternity/adoption
   2. Military service
   3. Union business and conventions
   4. Educational advancement
   5. Travel
   6. Personal
   7. Other
C. Process for requests
   1. Length of service
   2. Special circumstances
   3. Time limits
   4. Other
D. Accrual of seniority

XVI. Tuition Reimbursement
A. Definition of advanced education
B. Percentage paid by the hospital
C. Qualification
   1. Length of service
   2. Job-related education programs
   3. Personal interest education programs
D. Return to work requirements

XVII. Nurse-Management Committees
A. Types of joint committees
   1. Patient care
   2. Job description
   3. Evaluation
   4. Discipline/discharge
B. Purpose of committees
C. Meeting schedules
D. Selection of representatives
E. Role of committees
F. Activity and recommendations subject to the grievance procedure

XVIII. Insurance Plans
A. Health insurance
   1. Type of plan
   2. Scope of coverage
   3. Employer contribution
B. Health and welfare plan
   1. Through the hospital corporation
   2. Through the union

Outline of Sample Union Contract

  C. Retirement and pension plans
   1. Type of plan
   2. Percentage of employer contribution
   3. Eligibility requirements
   4. Vesting time
   5. Employee contribution plan
   6. Investment options
  D. Pharmacy discount
  E. Unemployment compensation
  F. Disability plan
  G. Occupational safety and health provision
  H. Other

XIX. Discipline and Discharge
  A. Warning process
   1. Verbal, written, or both
   2. Steps in warning process
   3. Limit on number of warnings
   4. Penalties attached
  B. Disciplinary action
   1. Procedure for taking action against nurse
   2. Notification in writing
      a. To nurse
      b. To union
   3. Time limits
   4. Joint determination
  C. Discharge requiring no warning
   1. Specify actions
   2. How is policy determined and approved
   3. Time limits for penalty of discharge
   4. Process
      a. Suspension during investigation
      b. Use of grievance procedure
  D. Discharge
   1. Reasons for discharge
      a. Violations of specific rules
         1. Determined by whom
         2. Approved by whom
      b. Violation of jointly determined code of ethics
   2. Types of discharge
      a. With notice
      b. Without notice

3. Hospital right to discharge
   a. Subject to union review
   b. Subject to grievance procedure
   c. Other
4. Notice and explanation of discharge
   a. Written explanation
   b. Notify union
E. Reinstatement
   1. Seniority rights and original position
   2. Back pay
   3. Combination

XX. Bulletin Boards
   A. Number and specific location
   B. Posting of union notices

XXI. Grievance and Arbitration Process
   A. Role of grievance committee
      1. Representation in meetings with hospital management
      2. Investigation of complaints
         a. With pay
         b. Without pay
         c. Requests for time off
      3. Other
   B. Definition of a grievance
      1. Violation of contract
      2. Past practices and existing law
      3. No limitation
      4. Other
   C. Time limits for filing grievances
   D. Steps in filing of grievances
   E. Description of arbitration procedure
      1. Process to select arbitration process
      2. Process to select arbitrators
      3. Payment of arbitration costs
      4. Role of the arbitrator
      5. Other

XXII. No Strike—No Lock-Out
   A. No strike provision
   B. Sympathy strike provision
   C. No lock-out provision

Outline of Sample Union Contract

   D. Use of grievance procedure and arbitration
   E. Wildcat strikes

XXIII. Duration of the Contract
   A. Length of the contract
   B. Automatic extension agreement
   C. Re-opener provisions
     1. Time frame
     2. Topics for discussion
     3. Notification requirements

Appendix C
Sample Employment Agreement (between group practice and C.R.N.A. employee)

This Agreement made this _____ day of _____, 19 ___, between _____, (hereinafter "Employer") and _____, C.R.N.A. (hereinafter "Employee").

WITNESSETH

Whereas, the Employer desires to employ the Employee to render anesthesia services;

Whereas, the Employee is licensed to practice nursing in the State of _____, duly qualified to practice nurse anesthesia, and desires employment as a nurse anesthetist;

Now, therefore, in consideration of the mutual covenants and agreements hereinafter contained, it is understood and agreed by and between the parties hereto as follows:

1. **Employment.** The Employer hereby employs the employee and the Employee hereby accepts employment upon the terms and conditions hereinafter set forth.

2. **Services.** Employee agrees to devote his/her working time and attention to practice as a nurse anesthetist for Employer, at such location or locations as shall be mutually agreed. In addition to ordinary working hours, Employee shall be available for emergency services on an on-call basis on holidays, evenings, and weekends as arranged between the parties.

3. **Term.** This Agreement shall remain in full force and effect for the period of _____ years from the date of execution and shall continue for successive terms of like duration unless either party shall within ninety (90) days of termination of the original or any subsequent term, give notice of its intent to terminate the then current term. However, the Employer shall have the right to terminate this Agreement for cause at any time upon thirty (30) days written notice for one of the following reasons only:

a. Finding of guilty for a crime involving moral turpitude;
b. Gross or culpable professional negligence; or
c. Death of Employee, or disability of Employee lasting longer than twelve (12) months.

In addition, this Agreement shall automatically terminate in the event that Employee shall have his/her license to practice nursing suspended or revoked by the State of _____, or any agency thereof, or

Sample Agreement: Group Practice and C.R.N.A.

his/her certification to practice nurse anesthesia suspended or revoked by the Council on Recertification of Nurse Anesthetists or other nationally recognized body. Employee shall have the right to terminate this Agreement for cause at any time for nonpayment of compensation. Any written notice required to be given by this paragraph shall be deemed to have been given upon deposit of such written notice in the U.S. mail, postage prepaid, or upon personal delivery.

4. **Compensation.** For all services rendered by the employee under this agreement, the employer shall pay the employee a salary of $_____ per year payable in equal semimonthly installments on the 15th day and the last day of each month. This amount shall be in consideration of work of 35 hours or for each hour worked on holidays or weekends, employee shall receive overtime pay in the amount of one and one-half times his/her regular hourly rate.

5. **Vacation and sick time.** Employee shall be entitled to 15 days vacation and 12 days sick leave per year. Vacation time and sick leave shall accrue as of the date of execution of this Agreement at the rate of 1-¼ days and 1 day per month, respectively, and both vacation time and sick leave shall accumulate from year to year. In addition, Employee shall be entitled to leaves to attend professional seminars, educational programs, and the like without loss of compensation upon the approval of the employer.

6. **Health and disability insurance.** Employer shall provide employee with and shall pay premiums on standard medical and disability policies of insurance, with benefits payable to Employee or his/her designated beneficiary, in the event of his/her illness, hospitalization, or disability in accordance with terms of said policies.

7. **Facilities.** Employer shall provide appropriate facilities and equipment to enable Employee to perform his/her duties hereunder.

8. **Malpractice insurance.** Employer shall purchase and maintain in force during the term of this Agreement for the benefit of the Employee comprehensive professional liability and general liability insurance with minimum limits of $100,000 per occurence and $300,000 aggregate, which is written on an occurence basis. The employer shall deliver a certificate of insurance to the Employee as evidence of this insurance.

9. **Expenses.** In the event that the Employee is requested to report to a location other than one to which there has been mutual agreement, the Employer shall reimburse the Employee for reasonable transportation costs to and from such location.

10. This Agreement shall be deemed to have been made and shall be governed by and construed under the laws of the State of _____.

In witness whereof, the Employer and the Employee have executed this Agreement as of the day and year first written above.

Employer
_____

Attest
_____

Employee
_____

Appendix D
Sample Employment Agreement (between hospital and independent contractor C.R.N.A.)

This Agreement, made this _____ day of _____, 19 _____, between _____ Hospital, a _____ corporation (hereinafter referred to as "Hospital") and _____ C.R.N.A. (herinafter referred to as "Nurse Anesthetist").

WITNESSETH

Whereas the Hospital is the owner and operator of a hospital located in _____, in which anesthesia services are rendered;

Whereas, the Nurse Anesthetist (a) is licensed as a registered nurse in the State of _____, (b) is duly qualified to practice nurse anesthesia, and (c) has current certification from the Council on Certification of Nurse Anesthetists, the Council of Recertification of Nurse Anesthetists, or another nationally recognized body; and

Whereas, the parties desire to provide a full statement of their agreement in connection with the employment of the Nurse Anesthetist in the Hospital during the term of this Agreement.

Therefore, in consideration of the mutual covenants and agreements of this contract, it is understood and agreed by and between the parties hereto as follows:

1. The Hospital hereby employs the Nurse Anesthetist and the Nurse Anesthetist hereby accepts employment on the terms and conditions set forth herein. The Nurse Anesthetist shall be certified by the Council on Certification of Nurse Anesthetists, the Council on Recertification of Nurse Anesthetists or other nationally recognized body, and it is expressly agreed that continuation of this Agreement shall be dependent upon the Nurse Anesthetist's continued certification by such body.

2. The Nurse Anesthetist shall provide the following professional services to Hospital:

a. Rendering anesthesia services and performing such professional duties therewith which are customarily performed by nurse anesthesia personnel in the _____ area so as to serve effectively the needs of the patients of the Hospital.
b. In conjunction with the above paragraph (a), consultation with the attending physician upon request concerning the anesthesia services rendered as they affect the treatment and welfare of the patient.
c. Cooperation with and participation in, as indicated, formal programs of anesthesia training or education, if any, (such as residency programs and schools of nurse anesthesia).
d. Consultation with the Hospital concerning the level of charges for anes-

thesia services rendered by the Nurse Anesthetist, upon request of the Hospital.

e. Rendering anesthesia services in compliance with applicable statutes, rules, and regulations; Hospital policies, rules, and regulations; and in conformance with the professional standards of an applicable nationally recognized organization.

g. Cooperation with and participation in, as indicated, any quality assurance programs approved by the Hospital, which shall include a systematic review of the quality, safety, and appropriateness of anesthesia services as required by the JCAH.

3. In his/her administrative relationship, the Nurse Anesthetist shall be under the direction of the President of the Hospital or his/her designee, and shall be responsible to him/her for abiding by the administrative regulations of the Hospital. In performing the professional services hereunder the Nurse Anesthetist shall be under the overall direction of the Medical Director of anesthesia services at the Hospital or his/her qualified designee, or the physician or surgeon responsible for the patient's care.

4. The Nurse Anesthetist agrees to perform the services pursuant to paragraph 2 above during such hours as shall be mutually agreed to by the parties. In this regard, the Nurse Anesthetist shall be physically present at the Hospital an average of _____ hours, and shall be on call at such other times as arranged with the Hospital. It is understood that the Nurse Anesthetist's commitment to the Hospital shall be approximately a _____ commitment. The Nurse Anesthetist may practice nurse anesthesia at other institutions and locations so long as such outside practice does not materially interfere with the services required to be provided under this Agreement.

5. As the sole source of compensation hereunder, the Nurse Anesthetist shall bill and collect fees for services from his/her patients or those persons or third party payors responsible for services rendered to them.

5a. (Alternative paragraph) The Nurse Anesthetist shall file with the Medical Director of anesthesia services or the President of the Hospital a report of all anesthesia services rendered by him/her on a monthly basis. The Hospital shall charge for these services at the same time that charges for other services rendered to the patient are billed or collected. On or before the _____ day of each month, the Hospital shall pay the Nurse Anesthetist, the fees collected on his/her behalf for the preceding monthly period, and provide an accounting.

6. In the performance of the work, duties, and obligations undertaken by the Nurse Anesthetist under this Agreement, it is mutually understood and agreed that the Nurse Anesthetist is at all times acting and performing as an independent contractor practicing the profession of nursing and specializ-

ing in anesthesia. The Hospital shall neither have nor exercise any control or direction over the methods by which the Nurse Anesthetist shall perform his/her work and functions; the sole interest and responsibility of the Hospital is to insure that the service required by this Agreement shall be performed and rendered in a competent, efficient, and satisfactory manner.

7. The Nurse Anesthetist agrees to maintain professional liability insurance (commonly called malpractice insurance) at all times with minimum limits of $100,00 per occurance and $300,000 aggregate.

8. The Hospital shall make available, during the term of this Agreement, space designated for the department in which anesthesia services are rendered and in addition, shall make available such equipment, furniture, files, and supplies as is necessary for the proper operation of the department. The Hospital shall also assume the cost of any and all maintenance, repairs, inspections, accreditations, and licensures of said equipment. The Hospital shall retain all rights of title of possession and ownership in any and all equipment and supplies purchased or otherwise acquired for use in the department.

9. All applicable provisions of law and other rules and regulations of all governmental authorities relating to licensure and regulation of nurses, nurse anesthetists, hospitals, and the department of anesthesia shall be fully complied with by the parties to this Agreement; in addition, the Hospital shall also operate and conduct the department in accordance with the standards and recommendations of the JCAH and the bylaws, rules, regulations and administrative policies of the Hospital as amended.

10. This agreement shall remain in full force and effect for the term of 1 year from and after the _____ day of _____, 19 _____, and for successive terms of like duration unless either party shall, within 90 days of termination of the original term or any successive term, give written notice of intention to terminate this Agreement at the conclusion of the term then in progress. However, the Hospital shall have the right to terminate this Agreement for cause at any time upon thirty (30) days written notice for any one of the following reasons only:

a. Finding of quilty for a crime involving moral turpitude;
b. Gross or culpable professional negligence; or
c. Continual neglect of duty or violation of hospital policy, bylaws, rules, or regulations.

In addition, this Agreement shall automatically terminate in the event that the Nurse Anesthetist shall have his/her license to practice nursing suspended or revoked by the State of _____ or any agency thereof or his/her certification to practice nurse anesthesia suspended or revoked by the Council on Certification of Nurse Anesthetists or the Council on Recertification of Nurse Anesthetists or any other nationally recognized body. The Nurse Anesthetist shall have the right to terminate this Agreement for cause at any time for nonpayment of compensation. Any written notice required to be given by this Paragraph shall be deemed to have been given upon deposit of such written notice in the U.S. Mail, postage prepaid, or upon personal delivery.

11. This Agreement shall be deemed to have been made and shall be governed by and construed under the laws of the State of _____.

In witness whereof, the Hospital has caused this Agreement to be executed by its duly authorized officer and the Nurse Anesthetist has executed this Agreement as of the day and year first written above.

Hospital
By: _____

Attest

_____

Nurse Anesthetist

_____

Appendix E
Sample Employment Agreement (Between Hospital and Employee C.R.N.A.)

    This agreement, made this _____ day of _____, 19 _____, between _____ hospital, a _____ Corporation (hereinafter referred to as "Hospital") and _____ C.R.N.A. (hereinafter referred to as "Nurse Anesthetist").
Witnesseth

    Whereas, the Hospital is the owner and operator of a hospital located in _____, in which anesthesia services are rendered;

    Whereas, the Nurse Anesthetist (a) is licensed as a registered nurse in the State of _____, (b) is duly qualified to practice nurse anesthesia, and (c) has current certification from the Council of Certification of Nurse Anesthetists or the Council on Recertification of Nurse Aneshtetists or another nationally recognized body; and

    Whereas, the parties desire to provide a full statement of their agreement in connection with the employment of the Nurse Anesthetist in the Hospital during the term of this Agreement.

    Therefore, in consideration of the mutual covenants and agreements of this contract, it is agreed by and between the parties as follows:

    1. **Employment.** The Hospital hereby employs the Nurse Anesthetist and the Nurse Anesthetist hereby accepts employment on the terms and conditions set forth herein.

    2. **Services.** The Nurse Anesthetist agrees to devote his/her working time and attention to practice as a nurse anesthetist for the Hospital and to render such professional services as are customarily performed by nurse anesthesia personnel in the _____ area so as to serve effectively the needs of the patients of the Hospital. In addition to working ordinary hours, the Nurse Anesthetist shall be available for emergency services on an on-call basis at such times as arranged between the parties.

    3. **Term.** This Agreement shall remain in full force and effect for the period of _____ years from the date of execution and shall continue for successive terms of like duration unless either party shall within ninety (90) days of termination of the original or any subsequent term, give notice of its intent to terminate the then current term. However, the Hospital shall have the right to terminate this Agreement for cause at anytime upon thirty (30) days written notification for any one of the following reasons only:

a. Finding of guilty for a crime involving moral turpitude;
b. Gross or culpable professional negligence; or
c. Continual neglect of duty or violation of Hospital policy, bylaws, rules, and regulations.

In addition, this Agreement shall automatically terminate in the event that the Nurse Anesthetist shall have his/her license to practice nursing suspended or revoked by the State of _____ or any agency thereof, or his/her certification to practice nurse anesthesia suspended or revoked by the Council on Certification of Nurse Anesthetists or the Council on Recertification of Nurse Anesthetists or other nationally recognized body. The Nurse Anesthetist shall have the right to terminate this agreement for cause at any time for nonpayment of compensation.

Any written notice required to be given by this paragraph shall be deemed to have been given upon deposit of such written notice in the U.S. mail, postage prepaid, or upon personal delivery.

4. **Compensation.** For all services rendered by the Nurse Anesthetist under this Agreement, the Hospital shall pay the Nurse Anesthetist a salary of $ _____ per year payable in equal semimonthly installments on the 15th day and the last day of each month. This amount shall be in consideration of work of 35 hours per week Monday through Friday at such times as arranged between the parties. For each hour worked in excess of 35 hours or for each hour worked on holidays or weekends, the Nurse Anesthetist shall receive overtime pay in the amount of 1½ times his/her regular hourly rate.

5. **Vacation and Sick Time.** The Nurse Anesthetist shall be entitled to 15 days vacation and 12 days sick leave per year. Vacation time and sick leave shall accrue at the rate of 1-¼ days and 1 day per month, respectively, as of the date of execution of this Agreement, and both vacation time and sick leave shall accummulate from year to year. In addition, the Nurse Anesthetist shall be entitled to leaves to attend professional seminars, educational programs, and the like without loss of compensation upon the approval of the Hospital.

6. **Health and Disability Insurance.** The Hospital shall provide the Nurse Anesthetist with and shall pay premiums on standard medical and disability policies of insurance, with benefits payable to the Nurse Anesthetist or his/her designated beneficiary, in the event of his/her illness, hospitalization, or disability in accordance with terms of said policies.

7. **Facilities.** The Hospital shall provide appropriate facilities and equipment to enable the Nurse Anesthetist to perform his/her duties hereunder.

8. **Malpractice Insurance.** The Hospital shall purchase and maintain in force during the term of this Agreement for the benefit of the Nurse Anesthetist comprehensive professional liability and general liability insurance with minimum limits of $100,000 per occurrence and $300,000 aggregate which is written on an occurrence basis. The Hospital shall deliver a certificate of insurance to the Nurse Anesthetist as evidence of this insurance.

Sample Agreement: Hospital and Employee C.R.N.A.

9. This Agreement shall be deemed to have been made in and shall be governed by and construed under the laws of the State of _____.

In witness whereof, the Hospital has caused this Agreement to be executed by is duly authorized officer and the Nurse Anesthetist has executed this Agreement both as of the day and year first written above.

                        Hospital
                        By: _____

Attest

_____

                        Nurse Anesthetist
                        _____

_____

Appendix F
Sample Employment Agreement (Between Hospital and Group Practice of which C.R.N.A. Is an Employee)

This agreement made this _____ day of _____, 19___, between _____ Hospital, a _____ corporation (hereinafter "Hospital") and _____ a group practice (hereinafter "Company").

Witnesseth

Whereas, the Hospital is the owner and operator of a Hospital in _____ in which there is located a Department of Anesthesia; and

Whereas, _____, is a _____ which employs nurse anesthetists who are licensed to practice nursing in the State of _____ and who are duly qualified to practice nurse anesthesia (hereinafter "Professional Employee");

Whereas, the parties desire to provide a full statement of their respective responsibilities in connection with the operation of the said Department of Anesthesia during the term of this Agreement;

Now, therefore, in consideration of the mutual covenants and agreements hereinafter contained, it is understood and agreed by and between the parties hereto as follows:

1. The Company hereby agrees to provide professional and administrative services to the Hospital's inpatients and outpatients in the Department of Anesthesia and the Hospital agrees to retain the Company to provide such services subject to the terms and conditions set forth herein.

2. In consideration of the funds and efforts the company intends to invest in performing under this Agreement, the Company shall have the exclusive right during the term of this Agreement to provide anesthesia services to the Hospital's patients; provided, however, that the right herein conferred on the Company shall not preclude present Medical Staff Members or other personnel who have been granted limited anesthesia privileges from providing anesthesia services to their private patients. The Hospital is desirous of an exclusive arrangement with the Company in order to maintain a high standard of anesthesia services, and recognizes that such an arrangement will facilitate overall surveillance of and scheduling in the Department and promote continuity of patient care.

3. The Company shall provide the following professional services to the Hospital in the Department:

a. Rendering all anesthesia services and performing such professional duties therewith which are customarily performed by nurse anesthesia personnel in the _____ area so as to serve effectively the needs of the patients at the hospital.

Sample Agreement: Group Practice and C.R.N.A. 153

b. In conjunction with the above paragraph (a), consultation with the attending physician, upon request, concerning the anesthesia services rendered as they affect the treatment and welfare of the patient.
c. Cooperation with and participation in the development of formal programs of anesthesia training of education such as residency programs, if any.
d. Evaluation of and recommendations for the purchase of major equipment, new or replacement, for the Department.
e. Advice and assistance in the development of the Department as appropriate to the Hospital's plan for development.
f. Consultation with the Hospital concerning the level of charges for anesthesia services in the Department, upon request of the Hospital.
g. Rendering anesthesia services in compliance with applicable statutes, rules, and regulations; Hospital policies, rules, and regulations; and in conformance with the professional standards of an applicable nationally recognized organization.
h. Participation in a Quality Assurance Program as indicated, which shall include a systematic review of the quality, safety, and appropriateness of anesthesia.

In their administrative relationships, the Professional Employees shall be under the direction of the President of the Hospital or his/her designee, and shall be responsible to him/her for abiding by the administrative regulations of the Hospital. In performing the professional services under the foregoing paragraph, the Professional Employees of the Company shall be professionally accountable to the Director of the Department.

4. The Company agrees to perform the services pursant to paragraphs 3 and 4 on a _____ (_____) hour, _____ (_____) days per week basis.

5. The Professional Employees of the Company shall be certifed by the Council on Certification of Nurse Anesthetists or the Council on Recertification of Nurse Anesthetists or some other nationally recognized body. It is expressly agreed that continuation of this Agreement shall be dependent upon such continued certification or recertification.

6. The Company shall establish all charges for anesthesia services rendered in the Department; these charges shall be billed and collected by the Company. In establishing such charges, the Company shall seek the counsel and recommendations of the Hospital. As the sole source of compensation hereunder, the Company shall look exclusively to its patients, or to those persons or third party payers who are responsible for services rendered to them.

7. The Company agrees at all times to maintain professional liability and general liability insurance (commonly called malpractice insurance)

covering it and each Professional Employee in the amounts of not less than $100,000 per occurrence and $300,000 annual aggregate or such higher amounts as shall be mutually agreed.

    8. The medical records of patients of the Hospital who are provided anesthesia services hereunder shall at all times be treated as confidential. Access and release of such medical records or any information shall be in accordance with the Hospital's policies.

    9. In the performance of the work, duties and obligations undertaken by the Company and its Professional Employees under this Agreement, it is mutually understood and agreed that the Company and its Professional Employees are at all times acting and performing as independent contractors and exercising their own independent professional judgment. The Hospital shall neither have nor exercise any control or direction over the methods by which the Company or its Professional Employees or others under their control shall perform their work and functions; the sole interest and responsibility of the Hospital is to provide overall surveillance of the Department and of services covered by this Agreement. All applicable provisions of law and other rules and regulations of any and all governmental authorities relation to licesure and regulation of nurses, nurse anesthetists, and hospitals and to the operation of the Department shall be fully complied with by all parties hereto; in addition, the parties shall also cooperate and conduct the department in accordance with the standards and recommendations of the JCAH, the State Department of Public Health, and the Bylaws, Rules, and Regulations of the Hospital as amended.

    10. The Hospital shall make available, during the term of this Agreement, space designated for the Department, and in addition, shall make available such equipment and supplies as mutually agreed is necessary for the proper operation of the Department. This shall not constitute any waiver or delegation by the Hospital of the right to purchase, lease, sell, or otherwise acquire, dispose, or replace capital equipment for said Department, except that in so doing, the Hospital shall first consult with the Company as to the necessity of doing so. The Hospital shall also assume the cost of any and all maintenance, repairs, inspections, accreditations, and licensures of said equipment.

    11. This Agreement shall remain in full force and effect for the period of _____ years from the date of its execution and shall be automatically renewed for successive terms of like duration unless either party shall, within ninety (90) days of termination of the term, or any successive term give written notice of its intent to terminate this Agreement at the conclusion of the then current term. The Hospital shall have the right to terminate this Agreement or any continuation thereof for cause upon thirty (30) written notice to the Company for any one of the following reasons:

Sample Agreement: Hospital and Group Practice

a. Finding of guilty for a crime involving moral turpitude of any person performing services pursuant to this Agreement;
b. Gross or culpable professional negligence by any person performing services pursuant to this Agreement; or
c. Continual neglect of duty or violation of Hospital or Medical Staff policies, Bylaws, Rules, and Regulations by any person performing services pursuant to this Agreement.

14. This Agreement shall be deemed to have been made and shall be construed and interpreted in accordance with the laws of the State of _____.

In witness whereof, the Hospital has caused this Agreement to be executed by its duly authorized officer and the Company has caused this Agreement to be executed by its duly authorized representative as of the day and year first above written.

_____Hospital
By: _____
_____ Hospital
By: _____
Attest
_____

Case Index

Ascher v. Gutierrez, 41–42
Austin v. The Regents of the University of California, 65

Beausoleiu v. Providential Sisters of Charity, 71, 82
Burne v. Belinkoff, 44–45

Calvero v. Franklin General Benev. Soc., 87, 92
Canterbury v. Spence, 70–71
Capili v. Mott, 100
Chalmers-Francis v. Nelson, 2–3
Clark v. Gibbons, 75
Cobbs v. Grant, 34, 37

Darling v. Charleston Community Hospital, 88, 92

Eng v. Valley Memorial Hospital, 88
Ewen v. Baton Rouge General Hospital, 54

Flanagan v. General Hospital, 55

Garland v. California Society of Anesthesiologists et al., 94, 104
Garza v. Berlanga, 46
Gravis v. Physicians and Surgeons Hospital of Alice, 35
Group Health Cooperative of Puget Sound v. Group Health C.R.N.A. Employees Group, 103–104

Hawkins v. McCluskey, 42–43
Herbert v. Travelers Indemnity Co. (1966), 87
Herbert v. Travellers Indemnity Co. (1969) 73
Herbert v. Woman's Hospital Foundation, 101
Hodgson v. Golden Isles Nursing Home, 94, 104
Holmes v. Gamble, 67–69
Hughes v. J. Jefferson Parish Hospital, 100

Jones v. Harrisburg Polyclinic Hospital, 54

Karrigan v. Nazareth Convent & Academy, Inc., 50

Lathon v. Hadley Memorial Hospital, 87, 92
Los Alamos Medical Center, Inc. v. Coe, 44

Mackey v. Greenview Hosp. Inc., 56–57
Magit v. Board of Medical Examiners, 3
Martin v. Stratton, 78–79
Marvulli v. Elshire, 85
Mayor v. Dawsett, 74–75
McCarl v. Commonwealth of Pennsylvania State Board of Nurse Examiners, 22–25
McConnell v. Williams, 85
McKenna v. Cedars of Lebanon Hospital, 57
McKinney v. Nash, 73–74
Meduba v. Benedictus Hospital, 87, 92
Mohr v. Jenkins, 52
Mulder v. Parke Davis & Co., 51

Napier v. Northern, 36, 79
Northern Insurance Co. of New York v. Superior Court, 42

Penderson v. Dumouchel, 88–89
Pugsley v. Privette, 33–34

Quintal v. Laurel Groves Hospital, 87, 92

Ramsland v. Shaw, 75–76
Regas v. Argonaut Southern Insurance Co. et al., 45–46

Sanzari v. Rosenfeld, 50
Sauro v. Shea, 107
Schneider v. Albert Einstein Medical Center, 46–47
Seaton v. Rosenberg, 106–107
Senero v. Haas, 72
Sesselman v. Muhlenberg Hospital, 85–86
Southeastern Kentucky Baptist v. Bruce, 48–49
Stevens v. Union Memorial Hospital, 53–54
Swanson v. St. John's Lutheran Hospital, 96

Tighe v. Commonwealth of Pennsylvania, State Board of Nurse Examiners, 22

Wagner v. Kaiser Foundation Hospital, 109–110
Webb v. Jones, 44
Wiles v. Myerly, 49–50
Willinger v. Mercy Catholic Medical Center, 48
Wing Memorial Hospital Association and Massachusetts Nurses' Association v. The NLRB, 103

Younger v. Webster, 108

Index

Abandonment, premature termination of professional relationships during anesthesia and liability to, 41
Accreditation of hospitals, 26
Adult, consent by, 33
Adversary system, 8
Agency, 83–84
American Association of Nurse Anesthetists (AANA), 3
professional standards of, 43–44
Anesthesia
brachial block, 78–79
dental, 107–108, 119
epidural, 76
obstetric, 112–113
regional. See Regional anesthesia
safety of, 61–62
spinal. See Spinal anesthesia
Anesthesia accidents, 59–65
first recorded death from anesthesia, 59–60
nerve damage, 67–69
obstetric, 64–65
preventable, 62–64

Anesthesia equipment
duty for maintenance of, 42–43
manufacturers' instructions on use of, as evidence of standard of care, 50–51
for regional anesthesia, 80
Appeals, 11
Appellate courts, 7, 11
Arbitration, 12
Assault, 31
Attorney General opinions, 13, 29–30

Bargaining units, 102–103
Barton, Sally, 104
Battery, 32
Bernard, Sister Mary, 1
Boards of registered nurses, suspension and revocation of license by, 21–25
"Borrowed servant" theory, 84
Brachial block, 78–79
Breaches of contract, 97
"But for" test to establish causation, 45

159

"Captain of the ship" doctrine, 85
Cardiac arrest
   during anesthesia for eye surgery, 111–112
   causes of, 62
   res ipsa loquitur doctrine in cases of, 53–54
Causation in malpractice actions, 45–46
Charts in regional anesthesia cases, 81
Civil rights laws, 94–96
Closing statement, 10
Collective bargaining, 102–103
"Common knowledge" rule, 49–50
Common law, 5–6
Comparative negligence, 56
Compensatory damages, 47
Complaint, 8
Consent, 31–37
   express, 32
   implied, 32
   informed, 34–37
   for surgery and anesthesia, 31–32
   who may give, 33
   withdrawal of, 33–34
Consideration in contract law, 97
Constitution of the United States, 6
Constitutions, state, 6
Contracts, 96–101
   breaches of, 97
   defined, 96–97
   elements of valid contracts, 97
   employment, 99–101
   exclusive, 100–101
   express, 98
   implied, 98
   written versus oral, 101
Contractual relationship, legal duty and, 40–42
Contributory negligence, 56–57
Cooper, J., 62, 67
Courts, appellate, 7, 11

Court system, 6–7
Crile, George C., 1

Damages, 47–49
   for breach of contract, 97
   compensatory, 47
   nominal, 47
   punitive, 47
   for wrongful death, 48–49
Defendant's case, 10
Defenses
   liability insurance and, 91
   to negligence, 55
Delivery room, presence of the father in the, 65
Dental anesthesia cases, 107–108, 119
Deposition, 9
Discovery, 9
Discovery rule, statutes of limitations and, 55–56
Dornette, 72–73, 76
Duty, negligence and, 40–43

Emergency care, good samaritan statutes and, 27–28
Employer-employee relationship, *respondeat superior* doctrine and, 83–84
Employment contracts, 99–101
Employment law, 93–104
   civil rights laws, 94–96
   contracts, 96–101
   labor law, 102–104
Endotracheal intubation in obstetrics, 65
ENT surgery, 113–114
Epidural anesthesia, 76–77
Equal Pay Act of 1963, 94
Equipment. *See* Anesthesia equipment
Evidence, 11–12
Exclusive contracts, 100

Index

Expert testimony (expert witnesses), 12
  exceptions to requirements for, 49–50
  qualification of, 49
  on standard of care, 43, 49
Express consent, 32
Express contracts, 98
Eye surgery, negligence cases involving, 109–112

Fair Employment Practice Act (Title VII), 94
Fair Labor Standards Act, 94
Fathers in the delivery room, 65

Gall bladder surgery case, 106–107
Good faith requirement in good samaritan laws, 57
Good samaritan statutes, 27–28, 57
Gross negligence, good samaritan immunity and, 28
Gynecologic surgery, 114–115

Health and Safety Codes, 25–26
Hodgins, Agatha, C., 1
Holding of the case, 11
Holmes, Oliver Wendell, 6
Hospitals
  accreditation of, 26
  liability of, 86–89
  state laws to regulate, 25–26

Identity of a patient, duty to verify, 42
Immunity, good samaritan, 27–28, 57
Implied consent, 32
Implied contracts, 98
INA Loss Control Services Inc., 60–61
Independent contractors, 84
  hospital liability for acts of, 86–88

Informed consent, 34–37
  for brachial block anesthetic, 79
  dental anesthesia cases, 107–108
  judicial interpretation of the need for, 35–36
  for regional anesthesia, 70–71
  for spinal anesthesia, 73–74
  statutes defining the law of, 36–37
Injunction as remedy for breach of contract, 97
Insurance, professional liability, 90–91
Interrogatory, 9

Joint Commission on Accreditation of Hospitals (JCAH), 26, 88
Jury, 10–11

King, J., 39

Labor law, 102–104
Larsen, 62
Lawsuits, 105–119 *See also.* Negligence
  brachial block, 78–79
  prevention of, 66–69
  regional anesthesia, 69–72
  spinal anesthesia, 72–76
Liability, 83–92
  agency relationship and, 83–84
  of hospitals, 86–89
  of nurse anesthetists, 89–90
  of physicians, 84–86
Liability insurance, professional, 90–92
License, suspension and revocation of, 21–25
Licensing of hospitals, 25–26
Literature as evidence of standard of care, 51–52
Locality rule, standards of care and, 44–45
Lumbar laminectomy, 110–111

Index

Magaw, Alice, 1
Malpractice. *See also* Lawsuits; Negligence
  interested parties in cases of, 39
  prevention of suits, 66–69
  statutes of limitations in cases of, 55–56
Manufacturers' instructions as evidence of standard of care, 50–51
Maternal mortality, anesthesia as cause of, 65
Medical literature as evidence of standard of care, 51–52
Medical practice acts, 25
Medical records as evidence, 11
Minors, consent by or for, 33
Monitoring patients
  eye surgery case, 109–110
  in regional anesthesia cases, 80–81
  of spinal anesthesia, 75–76
Multiple causation, 45
Municipal courts, 7
Mutual assent in contract law, 97

National Labor Relations Act, 102
National Labor Relations Board (NLRB), 102
Negligence, 39–47
  cardiac arrest case, 111–112
  causation in cases of, 45–47
  comparative, 56
  contributory, 56–57
  damages in, 47–49
  defenses to, 55
  dental anesthesia cases, 107–108, 119
  duty and, 40–43
  ENT surgery case, 113–114
  eye surgery cases, 109–112
  gall bladder surgery case, 106–107
  gynecologic surgery case, 114–115
  liability for acts of. *See* Liability
  lumbar laminectomy case, 110–111
  OB regional anesthesia case, 112–113
  orthopedic surgery case, 116–117
  pneumoencephalogram case, 117–118
  proving, 49–54
  in regional anesthesia, 71–72
  res ipsa loquitur doctrine and proof of, 52–54
  spinal anesthetic case, 108–109
  standard of care and, 43–45
Negligence suits, 8
Nerve damage, 67, 69
  after spinal anesthesia, 72–73
Neurologic deficits after spinal anesthesia, 72–73
"No duty" rule, 41
Nominal damages, 47
Nurse anesthesia
  Attorney General on, 29–30
  Joint Commission on Accreditation of Hospitals standards, 27
  legal recognition as a professional, 2–3
  origin of, 1–2
Nurse anesthetists, liability of, 89–90
Nurse Practice Acts, 14
  extracts from (table), 14–21

Obstetric anesthesia, 64–65
  epidural, 76
O'Rourke, Karen, 104
Orthopedic surgery, 116–117

Package inserts as evidence of standard of care, 50–52
Paralysis after spinal anesthesia, 72–73

Index

Physicians
  informed consent and, 35
  liability of, 84–86
Plaintiff's case, 10
Pneumoencephalogram, 117–118
Preanesthesia evaluation, 61, 66–68
  in regional anesthesia, 80
Precedent, concept of, 5–6
Prevention of suits, 66–69
Professional liability insurance, 90–92
Professional negligence. See Negligence
Professional relationships, legal duty and, 40–42
Professional standards of care, 43–44
Punitive damages, 47

Rapport with the patient, 66
Reasonable person standard, negligence and, 39
Regional anesthesia, 69–72, 112–113
  informed consent for, 70–71
  negligence in, 71–72
  prevention and defense of lawsuits from, 79–81
Regulations, 13
  voluntary, 26–27
Res ipsa loquitur, doctrine of, 52–54
  in regional anesthesia cases, 71–72
  in spinal anesthesia cases, 74–75, 108–109
Respondeat superior, doctrine of, 83–84
  hospital liability and, 86–87
Response, 8–9
Revocation of license, 21–25

Settlements, 9–10
  liability insurance and, 91

Specific performance as remedy for breach of contract, 97
Spinal anesthesia, 72–76, 108–109
  informed consent for, 73–74
  res ipsa loquitur in cases of, 74–75
Standard of care, 43–45
  "common knowledge" rule and, 49–50
  medical literature as evidence of, 51–52
  package inserts of drugs or manufactuers' instructions on use of equipment as evidence of, 50–51
Stare decisis, 5–6
Statute of limitations, 55–56
Statutes (statutory laws), 13
Substantial factor test to establish causation, 45
Supreme Court, United States, 7
Surgeons. See Physicians
Suspension of license, 21–25

Taft-Hartley Amendments, 102
Taylor, G., 62
Termination of professional relationship during anesthesia, 41–42
Testimony, expert. See Expert testimony
Textbooks as evidence of standard of care, 51–52
Trial courts, 7
Trials, 10–12

Unions, 102–104

Vicarious liability. See Liability
Voluntary regulations, 26–27

Wrongful death, 48–49
Wylie, W. D., 62

a
2 b
3 c
4 d
5 e
6 f
7 g
8 h
9 i
8 0 j